THE ALTERNATIVE
CHRISTMAS LETTERS

JOHN REDMOND

K7 PUBLICATIONS

For my wife and children

and

In memory of David, Mike and Terry,
fellow swimmers against the tide of
Parkinson's Disease, now no longer with us.

CONTENTS

PROLOGUE

I had reached the end of the line. It was December 2010, three months after I'd retired and exactly 15 years since my consultant had uttered those life-changing words: "I have no doubt you are in the early stages of Parkinson's Disease".

I had spent the last two nights shaking violently and sweating profusely in bed. I hadn't slept at all, watching the clock minute by minute as time stumbled excruciatingly slowly through the night. I had lost over two stone (over 12 kg) in weight because of the constant shaking and could only sleep with the help of drugs that reduced this. Due to potential side effects, I couldn't take enough drugs to keep me still for more than 12 hours a day.

My quality of life was at an all-time low. The only option left was deep brain stimulation, an eight-hour operation to attach an electrode to my brain, powered by a small battery sewn into my chest, much like a heart pacemaker. This allowed a small electric current to pass continuously through my brain, and was supposed to stop the shaking and reduce the amount of medication I needed. However, the operation was not without risks and there was no guarantee it would work.

Nevertheless, I knew I couldn't go on as I was. So, having told the kids where their inheritance was (just in case), I found myself, on a frosty winter's morning in January 2011, on a trolley being wheeled to the operating theatre at 8 am.

But I'm getting ahead of myself. The story of my Parkinson's Disease (PD) starts in a hotel room in South Carolina, in late May 1995. I was attending the fourth biannual conference of the American ECSA (European Community Studies Association) and had checked into the hotel, somewhat the worse for wear. I'd begun the day with a stressful drive to Heathrow airport, and had a long, tiring flight that I'd made easier to bear by drinking plenty of alcohol, which seemed like a good idea at the time. So, when I woke up the following day with my left arm shaking, I put it down to the aftereffects of the drink. But it persisted, even after I returned home. I eventually saw a consultant in December 1995 and the rest, as they say, is history. My struggle with Parkinson's is one of the recurring themes in what follows and provides a serious edge to what is meant to be a humorous book.

INTRODUCTION

The birth of Christ (Christ-mas) has been celebrated for over 2,000 years, though the earliest official records of this being celebrated on the 25th December only go back to AD 336, during the reign of Emperor Constantine of Rome, when the date was officially set at 25th December by Pope Julius 1. Over the years, many traditions have grown up to celebrate Christmas, but most of these are actually quite recent. For example, the Christmas tree did not come to Britain until the 1830s where it became an 'instant' tradition in 1841 when Prince Albert, Queen Victoria's German husband, had a Christmas tree set up in Windsor Castle.

Another Christmas tradition started in 1843, when the first Christmas cards were sent by Sir Henry Cole, a senior civil servant. History does not reveal if he included a Christmas letter with his cards, but I like to think he did, with a team of monks ready to make copies.

It probably went something like this:

Dear all,

Well, it's off to Balmoral for the family and me this Christmas. It'll be nice to see the Queen again. I haven't seen her since she gave me the knighthood as we've been on holiday to Europe for three months. We've visited many places…

six pages later…

While we've been away we had the castle decorated and our son…

four pages later…

etc., etc…

The snowbound image of Christmas in Britain owes more to Charles Dickens in the 19th century, and Hollywood fantasies of the 20th, than the reality of British weather patterns. More usually, it rains on Christmas Day.

Christmas traditions are thus largely a Victorian invention and owe much to Prince Albert. However, the simple and powerful message that the Christian Christmas offers, of peace, hope and goodwill, is much older and has much to commend it to all of us. Whatever its origins, tradition now dictates it is essential we do the same things, follow the same routine, and eat the same food. Christmas is about comfortable familiarity and spending time with the family, while trying not to argue. We do things at Christmas that we do very rarely, if at all, at other times of the year. Some traditions we share with everyone else, others are peculiar to our family, or just plain peculiar. These traditions change as we move through life. In my family's case, for example, they have included, and in some cases still do include, having takeaway pizza every Christmas Eve, the children watching 'The Snowman' and having 'The Night Before Christmas' read to them in bed, going to church, listening to the Queen's speech, eating Christmas dinner in the hall in front of the Christmas tree and taking turns to open presents, sat around the table after dinner, rather than ripping them all open before breakfast.

But my biggest personal tradition is my Christmas letter which goes to around 25-30 friends and relatives each year. These started as a spoof of the typed letters people send at Christmas, which tell the world about the great achievements of their wonderful offspring, holidays they have taken, and epic tales of how they decorated the kitchen and the spare bedroom. My letters took on a life of their own and became, in part, the kind of letter I was trying to poke fun at, but I have reined this tendency in and they remain largely what I intended at the beginning – a parody. Incidentally, we continue to receive such letters, even from some people to whom I send my parody letter. But many of my readership did get the joke and some have suggested I should share the letters with a wider audience – so here they are.

The 22 (and a half) annual letters, 1998-2020 inclusive, that appear here take in a whole range of activities and issues including pantomimes, holidays, family Christmases, Anthony Newley, the Eurozone, Latin and many other subjects. An important feature are the numerous opinionated flights of fantasy, which are largely fictional, although they may take a real event or activity as their starting point or may be a grossly exaggerated version of reality. In addition, the book contains jokes and quizzes. There is no story or plot as such. A few recurring themes do develop over time and give some sense of a story, but this is a book into which you can dip in and out at will. In addition, I blend elements of my autobiography into the letters, in which there are four overlapping themes:

1. My children and family life. Inevitably, they feature quite extensively in the book but mainly as digressions rather than central themes. At the time of my first letter in 1998, they were aged 17, 14, 9 and 6.

2. Growing up in a South Yorkshire mining village in the 1950s and 1960s. On the face of it, this sounds a potentially unpromising scenario but, in fact, I had a very happy childhood. Mining communities were very strong in those days based on sound values, respect for authority and strong moral principles. And, yes, I did play on the slagheaps and eat bread and dripping.

3. My life as an academic and professor. Academia is something of a closed book to the general public. I am unlikely to open it up completely but I do hope to give you some insights. I will say this, academia is one workplace where it is very appropriate to put up a notice that says 'You don't have to be mad to work here but it helps.'

4. Finally, this book is partly about my illness. I was diagnosed with Parkinson's Disease at the age of 42 in December 1995. So where does this book fit in on the spectrum of books by people talking about their disease or disability? Well, let me begin by

clearly stating what it is not. This book is not a catalogue of tips on how to cope with Parkinson's Disease. It is not a heroic tale of one man's struggle to come to terms with the condition. Nor is it a guide to how to live with Parkinson's or a ripping yarn about someone who refused to be cowed by the disease and went on to climb Mount Everest, or wrestle live alligators, or whatever their personal goal was, despite having PD. If you have PD then I send you my commiserations and good wishes, but I have no magic wand or bag of tricks to offer you. If you don't, then I hope to give you a greater awareness of the disease and to entertain you. If you were looking for Michael Parkinson's autobiography you are in the wrong place and need to look up "Parkinson" in the author index.

To reiterate, I incorporate PD, and my growing associated problems, into the letters, with the challenges becoming a little more dominant as the disease progresses.

The disease does progress and fighting it is like King Canute trying to push back the tide. Parkinson's is a variable, changing and slippery enemy against which you require constant vigilance in order to maintain some sort of quality of life. It is the gatecrasher who spoils your party, the burglar who steals your computer, the mugger who takes your wallet and the thug who kicks you when you are down. If this book does have a positive message, it is that you can only play the cards life deals you and there is no point in whining and feeling sorry for yourself. You just have to get on with it. You have to lower your expectations and live for today. There are some truly terrible diseases out there and PD is more manageable than most. Always remember, it is possible to be relatively content within the constraints of your illness and the only time you can be completely free of Parkinson's is when you are dead. With death as the alternative, having PD doesn't seem so bad.

So, there you have it. 'The Alternative Christmas Letters', a potpourri of a book with something for everyone and a rollercoaster ride of a read. Some of it is serious, a little depressing even, but much of it is humorous and guaranteed to put you in a good mood, glowing with the Christmas spirit in December, or glowing with a deep suntan (if you are reading the book on the beach) in July.

I hope you enjoy it whenever and wherever you are glowing.

Nil desperandum.

THE LETTERS

DECEMBER 1998

Welcome to our first Christmas letter. Christmas was not always easy in the past for my family. I particularly remember the winter of 1963, we were so short of money and fuel on Christmas Eve we had to saw off my uncle's wooden leg to burn while he slept in a chair. I can still remember the look of pained surprise on his face as he stood up to go and use the outside toilet, and keeled over into the fire. He kept us warm all night. He actually managed to climb out of the fire twice until my grandmother, showing great presence of mind, beat him unconscious with the poker. Times were hard but we were happy, and how we laughed! Not my uncle, obviously. But I digress...

We've resisted doing this for years but have finally succumbed, and so here is our very first Christmas Letter. Sorry I'm reduced to sending this rather impersonal note but I'm afraid I type much better than I write these days. The good news on the home front is we have moved house. The bad news is I am finding work increasingly a struggle due to the fact I have Parkinson's Disease. I'm now a shaker rather than a mover.

There are worse things out there, being eaten alive by a crocodile or getting stuck in a lift with Cilla Black, for example, but it does make life increasingly difficult. I was diagnosed at the end of 1995 and I've been taking medication ever since. The disease is controlled by drugs, or to be more precise, the symptoms are, although it is not an exact science. This is rather a depressing way to begin a letter primarily intended to wish you a happy Christmas, I suppose, but Anne thinks I ought to tell everyone I haven't told yet.

On the bright side, having PD did get me out of giving an inaugural lecture, a particularly barbaric ritual inflicted upon new professors at many universities. If you didn't know, I joined the professorial ranks in 1997. Not because I am particularly good at my job, but rather due to the fact that I had interviews for four chairs elsewhere and was offered one of them. The best way to get a chair at Edgbaston is to show them if they don't offer you one, you will go elsewhere.

The first two, which I didn't get, were at Leeds and Nottingham Trent. This left a bizarre few days in Hull being interviewed by the universities of Humberside and Hull, which were actually next to each other. Humberside was weird, I had already been offered the job at Hull and the external assessor, who has to be from another university, cried off at the last minute and was replaced very late by someone from Hull. This meant that the panel at Humberside must have known I'd been offered a chair at Hull earlier in the week. I also knew the assessor who cried off very well and I knew both the other candidates at Humberside.

It was all so incestuous and I decided fairly early on in the interview that I didn't want the job. I wasn't offered it and they eventually decided not to appoint anyone. I quickly decided not to take the job at Hull either, or rather, Anne did. Instead, I was straight on the phone to my head of department at Edgbaston with the 'good' news, and the rest, as they say, is history. Rather strangely, I turned down a lectureship at Hull ten years earlier when we lived in Sheffield. I'm probably not the University of Hull's favourite person! Nevertheless, the upshot of it all was my staying at Edgbaston on a promise and with three extra increments.

Despite all this excitement, we did manage a family holiday this year, albeit a rather unambitious, but nevertheless quite enjoyable, one in Wales. It was a sort of tour of a variety of Welsh towns while staying in pubs, the most bizarre of which was Tywyn, near Aberdovey. This was a seriously strange place with a desperately bleak seafront that gave a whole new meaning to the word desolate. There were two sad and isolated little amusement arcades, a transplanted country pub with garden that looked totally out of place, a number of faded and near-derelict Victorian houses, a 60's-ish, four-storey block of flats and, the *pièce de résistance*, a large field with eight sheep in it.

A field full of farm animals on the seafront must surely be unique. It wasn't clear whether the sheep were residents or on holiday, although they probably did live there as there was no evidence of buckets and spades or deckchairs. I had a photo taken in front of them just for the record. It's hard to believe anyone would willingly stay in such a place as a form of recreation, except perhaps a blind, workaholic sheepshearer, but then we were on holiday... This was not true of Caldey Island where both my family's religions are catered for: it is inhabited by Catholic monks who make chocolate!

We moved house earlier this year and therein lies a long and convoluted tale, sort of paradise gained, paradise lost and paradise regained. We found a house we really liked but couldn't afford, but we got more than we expected for our present house, the vendors of our 'dream' house came down a bit, and so we could afford it. We were all set up and I was just about to go away on business, when out of the blue we heard we were being dropped in favour of some neighbours, who coincidentally were using the same estate agent as our vendors!

So, feeling fairly depressed, I went off to a conference in the States, which was fairly dull and predictable although going over in the plane was certainly different. The flight seemed to be have been take over by Indians with turbans (Asian not Red, the Americans got rid of the Red Indians and stole their history), and men wearing red rugby shirts with Brains Bitter written on them, speaking Welsh. It was all slightly disorientating and I got completely confused while queuing at immigration and thought the Indian behind me was speaking Welsh – as far as I know, he might have been. It was by no means my first visit to the USA but I still can't decide if I like the place or not. At least I got into the country quickly, the immigration officials are usually very slow but were so taken by the idea of a beer called Brains, they fell about laughing and virtually waved us all through. If I do go to America again. I'm definitely wearing a turban and a rugby shirt with an unusual sponsor's name written on it.

On my return I went briefly to Brussels, a strange city in my opinion and an even stranger country, to which the number of my visits must now have reached close to double figures. What are you supposed to make of a country which can't decide which language to speak and is so obsessed with a statue of a little boy urinating, it has set aside a whole floor of a museum nearby to display the more than 300 costumes for him? The place always seems to be full of scaffolding and it rains, or snows, all the time. I was ostensibly there to interview someone in the European Commission about EU-Turkey relations, but Brussels is the place they invented the saying 'I'm only here for the beer' and so I visited a bar or three.

The beers are highly individual, often strong and served in a variety of special glasses. I once took a small party of students, including a Mr. Dong from Korea, known as Mr. Pong to our secretaries on account of his apparent tendency to eat raw garlic. There was no way you got into a lift with this man. It turned out that drinking Belgian beer also had an unfortunate effect on him. He had two glasses, began to act very strangely and disappeared into the night, not to be seen until the following evening. He was never quite the same again. It's lucky we were not in the bar with the stuffed horse on the stairs. That can be very disconcerting if you've had a few drinks and haven't seen it before. To be sure, it's a big enough surprise finding a horse in a pub when you're sober, although none of us would have been as surprised as the horse, I suppose.

The house saga had a happy ending because, lo and behold, when I got back home I received a phone call, on my birthday coincidentally, to tell us the new purchasers of the house we wanted had dropped out, and to ask if we were still interested? Six weeks later we moved in.

Houses are strange things. I remember a large house in the

centre of the village where I grew up, surrounded by a walled garden containing several apple trees. The house supposedly used to belong to a rich man, Mr. Napper, and possibly still did. No-one knew where he was and the house had been empty for years. What kept us out of the grounds and away from the apples was the alleged, and I think, occasionally real, presence of a gardener. He was there to tidy the garden and keep an eye on the property, and supposedly carried a stick and hated boys. Whether such a figure really existed I could not say. Certainly there probably was a gardener, but viewed from the comfort of advanced adulthood, it seems unlikely he was the stick-wielding, boy-hating ogre portrayed in the mythology of the six to 12 year old boys who played in the adjoining field. However, at that time we boys lived in terror of being chased by men with sticks and saw them everywhere. The shadowy figure in Napper's garden was supposed to have a counterpart who patrolled the Recreation Ground after dark, at the back of the village. Nowadays, of course, any man caught waving as much as a twig at a small boy would immediately be branded a paedophile and sent to the Esther Rantzen Clinic for the correction of dirty old men. But in those days your parents were much more likely to side with the man with the stick and even borrow his stick and give you a few extra whacks themselves.

Turning to the family, Angie only won one Nobel Prize this year (for wrestling) and continues to divide her time between her PhD in astrophysics and her hairdressing salon. Clare is still test driving for the Ferrari Formula 1 team but is hoping to move into accountancy later this year. Lizzie continues to train for the javelin at the 2000 Olympics and has nearly completed her book on fire-eating. James, aged 6, is doing his

GCSEs, whilst working in the evenings as a lion tamer to fund his hang-gliding hobby. Anne continues to combine being a 'supermum' with her two careers as a senior police officer and an airline pilot. She was found not guilty at the corruption trial back in April. So, a pretty uneventful year for the family.

Finally, just to fill you in with a few facts about Parkinson's. People think PD is about old people shaking but there is much more to it than that. It is caused by the brain cells that produce the chemical dopamine, which controls body movement, dying off and not reproducing. You can survive quite happily with a reduced amount until you reach a critical number of lost dopamine-producing cells and you've got PD. Usually, people aged over 60 get it, but five per cent of people diagnosed are under 40. I was 42.

Not everyone shakes, I don't much. My main problem is slowness and, without my drugs, lack of movement. It's not known what causes it, there are lots of theories but, it is degenerative and, at present, incurable, though they will find a cure, hopefully fairly soon, probably through gene research. It definitely is curable...eventually. So currently the symptoms are treated with drug therapy. You can control it pretty well for a long time, and I'm lucky that the demands of my job are such that I should be able to carry on working for some years. If I were a lorry driver or a brain surgeon, or indeed, a snooker player, I would be well-and-truly snookered.

And it should be remembered: there are three good things about Parkinson's Disease:

1. It doesn't kill you.
2. It isn't contagious, so you can't pass it on to your family.

3. It isn't especially painful for most people.

There is plenty more I could tell you but, although PD doesn't kill you, you can bore people to death talking about it, so I'll stop. Basically, I just have to get on with it.

And so, I will close on a happier note. We will spend Christmas in our new house for the first time this year and we are really looking forward to it. It should be a happy Christmas for us, and I wish the same for you and yours.

And, at this festive time of the year, remember the four stages of life:

1. You believe in Father Christmas
2. You don't believe in Father Christmas
3. You dress up as Father Christmas
4. You look like Father Christmas

Have a joyous and peaceful Christmas and a happy new year.

DECEMBER 1999

Hi! We have spent most of the year settling into our 'new' 200-year-old house. There is still lots to do but we like it here. We're only five minutes from the river, but high enough up not to flood, and 15 minutes' walk from the town centre. We are still on a main road, but the house is set back a little and is not too noisy.

Rather surprisingly, given the location of the house, we were burgled last February, but thankfully we didn't lose much. It's strangely unnerving being burgled. I suppose this is because it amounts to an intrusion into what is most people's ultimate safe place and sanctuary, their home. Our burglar was caught and it turns out our man was a career thief, released from prison on Friday, took the weekend off (even burglars need holidays), and was chased away by security guards whilst burgling the local college on Monday morning. During the chase he hid in our garden and must have taken note of our house, which he burgled in the afternoon. You have to admire his industry and persistence, if not his success rate. He is unlikely to get another chance though. A beneficial side-effect of having PD is that the house is rarely unoccupied, and most of the time I carry an alarm that is monitored 24/7 and allows me to call for outside help in case I get stuck or fall over.

Turning to the family, Anne has returned to nursing and works part-time in the Ophthalmic Unit at our local hospital. Angie (18) goes to the local technical college and plods on, while Clare (15) is taking her GCSEs, having passed music with an A* a year early. She continues with her flute and piano. Lizzie (ten) is in her last year at primary school and has just passed her Grade Two clarinet with distinction, to go with her Grade Two piano. We are still baffled as to where they get their musical ability from! Our son, James (seven), is mainly interested in football, computers and science fiction, especially Dr. Who.

Finally, despite my Parkinson's Disease, I continue to work at the university, commuting the 28 miles each way by car or, increasingly by train, although I find the train can be a little stressful. I recently emailed the following notice one afternoon to the departmental secretary to put on my office door.

I Don't Like Mondays

- 10.20 am Arrive Worcester Railway Station.
- 10.25 am Announcement that the 10.35, due at the university at 11.07, will today depart from Platform 2.
- 10.50 am The 10.35 departs from its usual Platform 1. They did tell us – at 10.49. We all have great fun watching the lady with crutches cross the footbridge for the second time. Oh, how we laughed!

- 10.51 am Train stops 400 yards from station. Line ahead blocked by broken down freight train.
- 12.30 pm Train returns to station. Train guard announces we are arriving at Worcester. This is followed by screams as passengers storm the guard's van and beat him to death with their tickets. OK, I made that last bit up.
- 12.40am All board another train which cannot leave yet because old train is in front of it. Passengers use explosives to blow up the first train in a desperate attempt to get to work by lunchtime. Well, they would have done if they had had any explosives.
- 12.50pm Discover there is no guarantee the train will get me to Edgbaston by 2.30 pm in time to do a few important things before my teaching.
- 12.55 pm Passengers now in open revolt: deliberately smoking in no-smoking compartments, flushing toilets while the train is in the station, not checking they have their personal belongings with them, and breaking their legs by deliberately not minding the gap as they get off the train.
- 1.05 pm I realise I may well not get to the university in time for my 3 pm lecture, and I have to get home.
- 1.06 pm I give up and go home.

Sometimes I think I'm living in a situation comedy.

(Much) later that afternoon, the train finally leaves Worcester.

I shall be in my office tomorrow between 10 am and 12.30 pm, and available for anyone who wanted to see me today.

Apologies.

––––––––––

In truth, the above is rather unfair. I quite like travelling by train and I particularly like the announcements.

My favourites include:

"This train is late due to following earlier trains." Do they normally overtake?

"This train is late due to an incident involving sheep at Bromsgrove." The mind boggles!

Said to me rather than announced: "There's a stiff on the line at Didcot Parkway, mate." Obviously a man who wisely chose to work on the railways rather than as a bereavement counsellor. But the old ones are always the best: "The train arriving at Platforms 1, 2, 3, 4, 5 and 6 is coming in sideways."

"British Rail apologise for the late arrival of The Rocket."

Talking of which, a relative doing our family tree discovered one of our ancestors was the third wife of George Stephenson, good old great, great, etc., great (step) uncle George.

Going back to PD, one of the perks (?) of having the disease, is that you get to join the PD Society. This is a registered charity and a very worthy organisation. Unfortunately, I'm a bit like Groucho Marx on this one, I don't want to join a club that will have me as a member. The problem is that many members of the PD Society are ill, they have PD! By definition, as I am relatively young and only recently diagnosed, most people with PD are older than me and their symptoms are worse than mine because their disease has had more time to progress.

I take the view that it is better for me to mix with 'normal' people, that is, people who don't have PD, and be dragged upwards, than to spend too much time with PD sufferers and be dragged downwards. Also, I don't have much in common with them. I don't care much for bingo, whist, daytrips to garden centres, watching TV quiz shows in the afternoon and keep fit for the over-80s. They tend not to like Jethro Tull, real ale and watching rugby.

Anne is very helpful on this as she makes little allowance for my PD, still expects me to wash up, mow the lawn and look after the kids. And I do still do these things, if a little more slowly than I used to, although I don't juggle or play the banjo. To be fair, I couldn't do either of those two things when I didn't have PD. We were recently introduced to a couple in which the man had PD, and his wife wrapped him up in cotton wool and did everything for him, helped him dress, fetched and carried things for him, peeled his grapes. The result was the man became what I call a professional invalid, and a PD bore, as in he could talk of little but PD. His symptoms were probably worse as a result, and he was certainly less independent.

None of this is intended to be criticism of the PD Society, which does exactly what it should for the majority of those with PD, and plays a vital role promoting and fundraising for research into a cure. It's just I'm not part of that majority and I'm not ready to get involved with the PD Society – yet.

However, I have joined the Young Parkinson's Group where young appears to have a rather broad definition and seems to mean simply 'not obviously old'. This group is a bit more relevant to my needs but there is still the problem of there being little else in common, other than having PD, and very few of us are still working. Part of the problem is that PD is a very individual disease and symptoms, problems and treatment vary across individuals. And then there are the side effects of the drugs. The NHS goes in for overkill and every drug comes with a list of potential side effects that covers virtually every possibility, from 'feeling drowsy' to 'growing facial hair and turning into Mr. Hyde'. To some extent, there is a grain of truth in that last one as the drugs can change your personality. For example, I'll bet you £20 you didn't know some PD sufferers have turned into chronic gamblers.

This letter is getting far too serious and so I'll stop now, another exciting instalment will probably follow next year. But finally, at the risk of pushing your level of excitement into overload, here is a Christmas joke.

Three men leave a Christmas party drunk, crash their car and are killed, and so find themselves waiting outside the pearly gates on Christmas Eve.

Saint Peter comes to the gates and says, "You three really ought to go downstairs, but as its Christmas I'll let you in if you can show me something Christmassy."

So, the first man pulls from his pocket a Christmas card someone gave him at the party and Saint Peter lets him in.

The second man pulls out his car keys, jangles them and starts singing 'Jingle Bells'. Saint Peter looks a bit dubious but waves him through.

The third man reaches into his pocket and pulls a pair of lady's knickers. Saint Peter is outraged and says, "What on earth have these knickers got to do with Christmas?"

"Ah," says the man, "they're Carol's."

It's the way I tell 'em.

Merry Christmas.

DECEMBER 2000

Well, here we are again, another year, another impersonal note. I'm getting a taste for writing these now. We are all well, including me, and we continue to plod on with the house. The floods have just subsided here. We were too high up to flood but the road between us and the river was closed for ten days and we had fun and games getting across the main bridge, sometimes in the back of an army truck.

Anne continues to nurse part-time in the Ophthalmic Unit at the main hospital in Worcester. Angie (19) still goes to the local technical college a couple of times a week but now works virtually full-time in a nursing home, where she used to volunteer. It paid off because they gave her a job. Clare (16) got a good set of GCSEs,11, and is now doing 'A' levels in Music, History, English Literature and Politics at the Sixth Form College, and impersonating a hippy. She passed Grade 6 flute and Grade 7 piano this year and played in Austria with the Worcestershire Youth Orchestra. She has also acquired a Saturday job in Boots and a boyfriend.

Lizzie (11) has started secondary school and is growing

fast. She's passed Grade 3 clarinet and Grade 3 piano, and is awaiting the results of her Grade 3 theory. But it's her drama school on Sundays, Stagecoach, that she's really into. She appeared in the children's chorus of a professional production of 'Joseph and his Amazing Technicolour Dreamcoat', at the Belgrave Theatre in Coventry for a week in June. James (eight) has also joined Stagecoach and is in their Christmas play, just for the parents, playing Joseph. He also auditioned for the school play and will be the 'chief angel'. According to James, the main perk of the job is he 'gets to boss the other angels around'.

John continues to work full-time at the university and is coping pretty well, probably better than last year, and has started going to conferences again. The new campaign, or new academic year as non-combatants prefer to call it, is well under way with students arriving from all corners of the globe – and other planets by the look of some of them. Several, I've no idea how many, new members of staff have arrived. I can't tell the difference between them and most of the new students to be honest. I just wander into the photocopying room and smile benignly at whoever's there. It seems to work. Actually, I don't envy the new staff teaching for the first time. I remember my early teaching all too well.

The first teaching I did was as a postgraduate student. It was very common for PhD, and even Masters, students to supplement their income by doing some teaching. My first classes were a couple of first year seminars at Cardiff, with about a dozen general economics students in each. This was followed by similar teaching when I went to do my PhD at Warwick. I remember nothing of this, but I do remember a story doing the rounds about one postgraduate tutor who walked into his first ever seminar, sat in a chair, leaned back against the wall he thought was there but wasn't, and fell flat on his back. However, I do recall some teaching I did at Coventry University (then Lanchester Polytechnic), which I got through my next-door neighbours who lectured there.

It was a tough audience consisting of around 50 HND Engineering students, who didn't want to be there, but had to do a 'liberal studies' course each year. This year it was economics. As you can imagine, being engineers, they did not hold economics or economists in high regard. In fact, I felt like Daniel going out to meet the lions each week. The students had little incentive to take an interest as there was no examination, and the only requirement was they attend 75 per cent of the course – I kept a register. The vast majority ignored me and just read books, which I could live with, but there were four troublemakers who tried it on in my second lecture, when they played cards throughout.

They were fairly quiet during the lecture and so I left them alone and waited until the end of the lecture, walked over to them and said quietly, "Playing cards does not constitute attending my lecture. I shall mark you absent." This was met with a chorus of complaints and cries of "You can't do that!" which I silenced by telling them to report me to their head of department. They never played cards or caused any trouble in my lectures again.

The role of teaching in a university lecturer's work is widely misunderstood. Lecturers regard it as a necessary evil, students regard it, wrongly, as their primary source of information. Parents think it is what they are paying for and university administrators ignore it, and forget it takes up a considerable amount of lecturers' time.

In fact, there are three elements that make up a lecturer's job: research, teaching and administration. Research is what academics want to do and what they think they are there for. Teaching is paid lip service, but the truth is academics are untrained amateurs and their teaching is offered on a take-it-or-leave-it basis. Lectures are purely a guide and students are expected to build on them by working in the library. Administration relates to things like course design and student admissions, and a whole range of committees dealing with often quite trivial academic matters. This is changing to some extent as training in, and assessment of, teaching becomes more widespread, but it is still research that determines who gets the job and who gets promoted.

These days, with several early retirements, I'm probably the most experienced teacher in the department. Certainly, I am the longest serving member of the department and so I'm allowed to be a little eccentric and appear to not really know anyone. Actually, I don't know anyone. In any case, universities are changing for the worse. Our Office Manager in newspeak, no. 1 secretary in proper English, is a case in point. She continues to jackboot her way around the department, firing larger and larger quantities of A4 paper from the hip, making more and more work, whilst simultaneously complaining she has too much to do. She could stop typing and making telephone calls for a start and read a bloody book, preferably one of mine then she might realise why I don't answer her memos. We also have a head of department who wants to love, and be loved by, everyone. He seems to have completely missed the point of being head of department. That is, this is the one chance you get in life to hate everyone and be able to do something about it, and disappear on a sabbatical afterwards. Our previous head is in Australia. It really is a mad world. Fortunately, I'm in a position to let most of it wash over me and worry about more important things, like Worcester rugby club.

It's amazing just how much I like rugby union, given I wasn't even aware of its existence for the first 11 years of my life. The only rugby I was vaguely aware of was rugby league (RL), because Doncaster, my home town, had a notoriously bad RL team. They habitually lost every game and finished bottom of the RL second division. The Dons, as they were called, were a joke, and I remember a TV documentary about them in the late 1960s. The programme showed their season as a build-up to a particular game, the home match against Hunslet, which came near the end. Hunslet usually finished second-from-bottom. It was a big game for Doncaster as it was the only one in the year which they stood the remotest chance of winning. As I recollect, they maintained their 100 per cent record and lost.

This blissful ignorance of rugby union was to be forcibly brought to an end in 1965, the year I passed my Eleven Plus, and started at the local grammar school. It was a typical northern grammar school where rugby union was the only winter game for boys, soccer was ignored. I can still vaguely remember my first contact with the game, standing shivering in line one cold September afternoon with several dozen other 11 year old boys, in my uncomfortably-new kit and clean, for the first and last time, boots. I certainly never cleaned them, it was bad enough having to bloody wear them. We were confronted by two sadists, cunningly disguised as games masters, who were to make those of us who didn't like or excel at the game miserable for the next five years.

We were only given relief when we reached the sixth form. The games masters, Reg and Rog(er), finally gave up on us, threw those of us who bothered to turn up a soccer football and buggered off back to the staff room, or went to coach their beloved First XV. To this day, whenever I'm in a group of around ten people, a similar size to a rugby scrum, I can still occasionally hear Reg's booming voice shouting out his mantra: Bind and heel, boys. Bind and heel.

For the next five years, from September until March, I was subjected to a torture called Double Games on a weekly basis. My mother could only be persuaded I needed a sick note on a limited number of occasions. In games lessons, sick notes were like gold dust to the boys and a necessary evil to the sadists. "Two broken legs? What sort of excuse is that, laddie? You could still play on the wing in that wheelchair." That was their answer to any injury, go out and recover on the wing. On a bad day there were so many real and feigned injuries that the wings were like a field hospital in a war zone. You needed an ambulance to ferry the recovering wingers up and down the touchline to keep up with play.

Some tried, mostly unsuccessfully, to forge sick notes but I had a better method. My mother never dated my notes and so, after they had been glanced at and scornfully binned, I would retrieve them for re-use at some future date. This gave some temporary respite, as did the two weeks in December when games were replaced by ballroom dancing lessons with the girls in preparation for the school's Christmas dance. This was torture of a different kind.

We stood in the line at the beginning of games, while Reg or Rog selected 15 victims to act as cannon fodder for the grinning trainee-sadists – the year's First XV – in the main game. When this ritual was over, the remainder heaved a sigh of relief and were organised into two or four scratch sides which competed on adjoining pitches, under whichever of Reg or Rog had drawn the short straw that day.

In reality, by mutual consent they didn't compete at all, just tried to get through the hour without hurting each other. Because I was biggish then, I was often selected as a prop in the Victims XV, which at least gave me somewhere to hide. But it was impossible to emerge at the end completely unscathed. Comparing how I was introduced to the game of rugby union with the experience of the current mini-rugby players, I wonder what the hell they thought they were doing. It was like being in the Dark Ages.

The beginning of my enlightenment came at a time when I thought my rugby days were behind me. In the upper sixth form to be precise, my last year in the school. There were Houses in such a traditional school and my house, Vermuyden (Red), had a problem. We were required to field a 15-man rugby team in the inter-house competition, and we only had 13 boys in the combined lower and upper sixth form. It was a case of all hands on deck. All 13 of us plus two fifth-formers, one of whom happened to be our only member of the school First XV. He was a precocious lad who went on to play for Yorkshire Boys. We took to the field against Brooke (Green), and thrashed them. We subsequently put another 50 points on Mowbray (Yellow). Then came the show-down with Warren (Blue) who were also unbeaten. Reg was their housemaster and two-thirds of the First XV were in their ranks.

We didn't win and were never going to, this isn't a fairy story, but we only lost narrowly and, marshalled by our precocious fifth-form fullback, gave them a good run for their money. I began to get some inkling of what the game was about, knowledge which fully developed when I went to university in Cardiff and discovered the Arms Park and Gareth Edwards.

I lived within walking distance of the Arms Park for most of my time in Cardiff. It was probably the golden era of Welsh rugby, and impossible to avoid getting caught up in the excitement that surrounded the (as-then) Five Nations Tournament. For two Saturday afternoons in the spring term, the streets of the city went quiet as people retreated to their televisions to watch the away games. For the two Saturdays of the home games, the city went mad and was awash with colour and singing drunks. The Scots were drunk and friendly in an aggressive way, the Irish were drunk and friendly in a humorous way, the French were drunk and friendly in a flamboyant way. I remember a gang of them lunched in the Students' Union one year and literally carried off one of the serving ladies to the pub afterwards, she didn't seem to mind. The English, I'm afraid to say, were just drunk and boring.

Attending the game meant you missed the wonderful commentaries of the legendary Bill McLaren. For many years, his commentary was as integral to a Five Nations international as the ball with which they played. I remember Bill's commentaries, not just for his obvious deep knowledge of the game, but for his masterly use of understatement and his generosity. No matter how horrendous the mistake, he found some mitigating circumstance. If a fullback knocked on when trying to catch a high kick, he was blinded by the sun, even when the game was played in thick fog or torrential rain. Or the ball was very slippery and like a bar of soap, or the player had been attacked from behind by an invisible crocodile at the critical moment, etc.

Bill would never say the player dropped the ball because he was a useless pillock, who couldn't hold on to the balls of a one-armed, legless scarecrow tied to a wooden stake. Moreover, I am pretty sure he wouldn't even have thought that. Furthermore, Bill transferred his generosity onto other people. So when a player did something good, Bill was absolutely certain they would be pleased down [name of player's club]way, or that those watching in the [name of player's club] clubhouse bar would be celebrating. Or they'd be excited in the service area by Junction 8 of the M5 Motorway where [name of player] always stops on his way to his holiday cottage in Cornwall in July.

Oh, happy days! But I digress. Have a happy and peaceful Christmas and I hope 2001 is a good year for all of us.

DECEMBER 2001

It's Christmas time again, time for another letter chronicling the Redmond family year! A brief comment to any male readers: this is the point at which to give the letter to your wife/mother/sister/dog/paper shredder so you don't have to read it, but can get the main points from someone else, so you can appear to have read it if we meet in the next year.

To be honest, I'm rather hoping this Christmas will be like the last one, very quiet with only my family. Last year's presents were pretty good, mine were predictable but what I wanted, not least because I'd taken the sensible precaution of buying a book on rugby and one or two other items myself and giving them to Anne to wrap. Daughter no. 2 had an electric guitar. After investing vast sums in her musical training in the past, I am now insisting she meets the deadline that I have set – of her 18th birthday - for her first Top 10 single. I am hoping she will eventually be interviewed by 'Melody Maker', or whatever is the equivalent nowadays, and tell them about the wonderful house she just bought her parents.

But the real joy was that after 20 years of bloody Barbie

and Sindy dolls, and the dreaded My Little Pony – I once spent the best part of an entire Christmas Eve putting a stable together for one of those ponies – I finally have a son old enough to get good presents. A six foot snooker table and Subbuteo last year; he even got to play with them a bit! Daughter number three got some horrible electronic dog, of which the cat was deeply suspicious.

Turning to the cat, she had a very traumatic start to 2001. At about 12.10 am on New Year's Day, the poor creature made the biggest mistake of its life. The kids had not shut the door properly and the cat appeared at my side a split-second after I'd lit a single-fuse mega-fireworks. It took my wife over an hour to get the animal out from behind the washing machine. I wanted to cut our losses, wall it in and go to bed, but was overruled and sent to my room in disgrace. Our previous cat, sadly run over after 4 months and just after he had finally realised the house and a toilet were not the same thing, had a much more sensible attitude to fireworks. He just sat on the window sill inside the house and watched them. It's a shame he didn't have the same attitude to moving vehicles. However, the cat made an even bigger mistake later in the year when she said, "Yes, alright then," to the old tomcat three doors away.

But to finish last Christmas. One of the highlights was a trip to Edgbaston, to the Alexandra to see the pantomime on Boxing day, although listening to Stephen Fry reading the first Harry Potter book on the radio driving there and back was better. The pantomime stars were pretty meaningless to me: Dirty Den from 'EastEnders' as Captain Hook, and some squeaky-voiced comedian who had a hit single with a song about songs that get on your nerves. At one point he said something about some people liking him and some not, I felt like shouting out that some of us didn't give a toss because we didn't know who the hell he was. To be fair, the sets, singing and dancing were first rate, although the story line was a bit weak. We were well entertained by the antics of a man in his 50s who took joining in to extremes. He was apparently without children, or possibly they were so embarrassed by him they sat elsewhere, a bar in Aberdeen perhaps. The kids thought, quite rightly, that the man was not very cool.

I've had a busy year. So much so, I've been less involved with the Young Parkinson's Group, well, youngish, I think I'm the second youngest and the only one still working. We've missed most meetings mainly because they involved talks about being ill and are held at Camp Saga, our base. It's conveniently next to a church, the cathedral no less, presumably so we can deal with sudden deaths – from depression, or boredom, or losing the will to live after listening to Jim's guitar playing. That is, Jim 'I've got PD but I'm very brave and can still do everything'. Wrong, Jim, you can't play the guitar, your musical ability is on a par with a one-legged, deaf and blind giraffe's Morris dancing skills. Returning to causes of sudden death, in Jim's case it will probably be from being beaten around the head by me, with the aforementioned guitar having finally cracked. More probably, as Jim's a clever-dick, (if this is the copy of the letter I've sent to my old friend Dick then no offence, mate!) by being trampled underfoot while trying to teach the giraffe to Morris dance.

The highlight of my year was a trip to the States in May, to a conference in Madison with a short visit to Washington beforehand. United Airlines are quite good on food, inflight entertainment, friendliness, just a bit weak on supplying airplanes. I arrived at Heathrow airport at 10 am for my 12.50

pm flight to Washington, to hear the flight would now be at 11.30 pm. A few of us protested a bit and I was eventually put on the 10.55 am to Boston, which I had to sprint (OK, walk quickly!) to catch. I flew on to Washington, arriving only an hour later than originally planned. Then the journey got really terrifying, a 45-minute taxi drive by a lunatic who had obviously lost the will to live and was probably working to earn money to pay for his funeral. He drove in the outside lane, with occasional swerves towards the concrete barrier dividing the road, well over the speed limit using one hand.

I always say the dangerous part of flying is the drive to the airport. However, I suppose I ought to be relieved I wasn't on Pan Am Flight 103 to New York and Detroit that year in the light of events at Lockerbie. (Lockerbie, in Scotland, is where, on 21 December 1988, the wreckage of Pan Am Flight 103 crashed after take-off from London, when a terrorist bomb on board detonated. A total of 270 people were killed.) I can personally confirm security on internal US flights was very limited. Washington was OK, I've been there before so I tried to see different things, the Holocaust Museum and Korean War Memorial. What a jolly day that was. Eventually, after they'd talked me down from the bridge and persuaded me things weren't so bad, and I'd had a night's sleep, I was ready for Madison.

It was not an auspicious arrival. As soon as we got off the plane it was taken out of service for a technical reason. It was raining, and I have to say Madison looked like the worst of Manchester on a bad day. The taxi driver whining about the rain didn't help. I got to the hotel about 7 pm, went to examine the pool and who should I bump into but one of my colleagues from Edgbaston! We Edgbaston boys know how to prioritise!

I think my first impression of Madison was correct, a one-horse town. My hotel was on the main square. I went out to get something to eat around 10 pm on Friday and...nothing. There were a couple of bars and no food anywhere. It was like a ghost town, even the one horse had gone. I wish I'd gone with him. I imagine the horses around here call Madison a one-man town.

I eventually had a pizza delivered, a large one and so enough to feed me and the horse. I went to find the horse, invited him up, and we watched a John Wayne film. The horse thought it was a philosophical film about man's treatment of horses.

I seemed to spend a fair amount of my time after leaving Washington watching John Wayne films, along with a sitcom about old ladies called 'The Golden Girls', and ice hockey. So many channels and so little to watch, although I must admit with 50 odd channels, just flicking through them kills half an hour. What I'd like to have seen was a cross between something like one of those home decorating programmes, a wildlife documentary and a magic show - it would have begun with 'Handy Andy' from 'Changing Rooms' sawing a badger in half.

Come to think of it, everyone had probably gone to bed early on Friday to prepare for the much-trumpeted-in-the-tourist-literature Farmer's Market, beginning at 6 am on Saturday. Right outside my hotel. This turned out to be a glorified car boot sale selling farm produce. Madison is the state capital of Wisconsin, the number one dairy state in the US, and so we had life-size plastic cows, men dressed as cows, cars painted as cows and a very large tent, with a display inside, painted to look like a cow. I had to walk through this to go to the conference. I asked someone about it and was told it wasn't usually like this. No, normally they have REAL cows, but couldn't today because of fear of spreading foot and mouth disease. This is supposed to reassure me? My God, they know how to give a cow a good time in Madison. It's nice to know the old British eccentricity is alive and well in our former colonies. It's not the guns that worry me when I visit the USA, it's the people holding them.

At last, it was time for me to leave. The horse came to see me off. Actually, I wish he'd come with me, I had to walk for half an hour between planes at Chicago. Minneapolis came and went. United upgraded me to business class on the way back but smashed up my case to keep me in my place. I got home to find myself locked out and had to wait for my 12 year old daughter to let me in. That completed being put in my place.

I arrived back just in time for the exam season. It was amazing this year. We put one of our German lecturers in charge and the examiners' meeting lasted less than an hour. As he read out the names one by one, I had to fight back a terribly strong urge to shout "Present!". This would have been totally politically incorrect, particularly as we had one of those all-day get togethers the following week, you know, where you bond with (or, in my case, are introduced to) your colleagues. Fortunately, it wasn't a completely boring day because we got a tour of our new building, and I didn't put my foot in it like I did on a previous occasion. Last year I spent the first session of the afternoon slagging off the content of the second session, to a former colleague, only to find he was the speaker for the second session. He'd left to develop the subject for the whole faculty. Whoops!

But back to buildings. I rather liked the old one. It was an ugly 1960's tower and we were on the 11th floor, but it did have certain advantages. One, the rooms were big. Two, students mostly couldn't be bothered to come and see you, and those who could, would only come when they had something urgent to see you about. Three, an office inside the building was the only place on campus from which you couldn't actually see it! As the longest serving member of the department, I did toy with the idea of barricading myself in my office and refusing to go, but knowing the way the University of Edgbaston works, I'd probably have been left to die there. Besides, I think the new building is pretty good.

We eventually got in it in early August, and it was eventually finished in November. It would have been nice to have finished it first, but moving in too early introduced an element of excitement to going to work. Would my phone and computer work? Which door would be open today? Would I be able to get out of the building at the end of the day?

My favourite feature is the lift. It talks and you can ask it questions like what is between the first and the third floor? 'Second floor'. And, what is at the bottom of the building? 'Ground floor'. It's not very good on ceilings though, although having said that, if it spoke Chinese and had £7000 then we'd probably give it a Master's degree. What I like the most about the lift is the little box with the floor number in because it also contains the words: Help is coming. It doesn't specify when, what for, and in what form, but I find it comforting to begin every working day knowing 'help is coming'.

The only downside of the new building, apart from the fact that the students seem to have found it, is our head of department, in a fit of misguided, egalitarian, political correctness, decided senior staff would not get bigger offices.

Offices would all be the same size. So, my office is a bit of a shoebox, although it has forced me to throw away piles of stuff I'd been hoarding for years. There has also been a general shortage of shelves. The response of School of Social Science, that "the academics have too many books" was amazing even by the university's normal standards. Perhaps we ought to throw them away when we've read them? Happily, I was on study leave from October which means I got to stay at home and tidy up after breakfast instead of going to work, every day rather than just on Tuesdays.

I suppose I ought to say something about my offspring. Angie is pregnant and we become grandparents in April. We're fairly relaxed about it, at least she made it out of her teens, she'll be just 21. Once you get to four kids, economies of scales set in, so I don't suppose we'll notice another one about the place. Clare is in the upper sixth and applying for university. She certainly has all the necessary credentials: her room is a tip, she has no money, she sleeps a great deal, is monosyllabic. She'll make a splendid student. Lizzie is on the verge of teenagerhood, and has been practising being horrible for some time. She's still into drama and spent two days filming in Bristol in the summer for a C4 kids' drama called 'Teachers'. She got paid £20 per day, which is a significant amount of money to a 12 year old. James has temporarily abandoned his training programme to prepare him for playing football, cricket, snooker and golf for England, so he too can tread the boards. In his case, as a munchkin in a one-week production of the Wizard of Oz at the Norbury Theatre, Droitwich. He had to do quite a lot, a little speaking and he had to sing three lines by himself. I thought he was pretty good for a nine year old. Anne continues... Actually, she just continues, she never stops. But I must stop. I've rambled on for long enough. Have a good and peaceful Christmas and a happy and prosperous year.

And remember. No matter how bad things get, there's always someone poorer, drunker, more tired, with an older car, and more children and cats to support than you – me!

Season's greetings.

DECEMBER 2002

Here we are, another year. 2002, a fairly dull one. I've not been to any exciting conferences and we've not had any major disasters – apart from Worcester's continued failure to get promoted to the rugby union premiership. I used to read about 2002 in my youth, when I was heavily into science fiction, and it's not lived up to expectations. Work is especially disappointing. The department is now officially wonderful, second in the Guardian league for our subject and received top marks when assessed for teaching and research. Our new head, who is even more determined to be loved than the old one, goes around thanking and congratulating everyone. Moreover, if my sources are correct, our old head has taken loving the department a bit too far by disappearing to Portugal on a sabbatical, and taking one of the female lecturers with him. Rumour has it they are planning a new life together in America.

In fact, with the exception of myself and the new head, all the professors in the department have wandered off, one is in

Portugal as I've said, one in the Far East, one seconded as head of something else, and one running the university's sociology degree. Our sociology department has a lemming-like tendency to self-destruct periodically. 20 years ago, it voted to close itself down because of internal disputes and disagreements. It seemed a bit extreme to me, but having reformed they have now done the same thing again. Unfortunately, they forgot to stop recruiting students, even though all the staff left, so we loaned them Mike. Personally, I would have thought that as an active Accrington Stanley supporter, he had enough tragedy in his life. On the other hand, he does seem to like drinking and has an interesting wife, so perhaps they want to study him.

I can identify with him on the football as I, too, used to support a team in the lower divisions. I supported Doncaster Rovers for six full seasons, during which they yo-yoed between the old Divisions 3 and 4. Come to think of it, I can see now why I switched to rugby union. I remember the first game I ever went to, in 1964, accompanied by my friend. It was spring and we were playing York, who were top of the league, but we went 4-0 up after 20 minutes and eventually won 4-3. My friend was in a daze and kept saying, "It isn't like this every week, you know." But I also remember the violence and football hooliganism rife at the time, even in the most unlikely of places. I went to Grimsby three times on 'football specials' in the 1960s, once by train and twice by bus. The first time, the Grimsby 'fans' stood on a bridge and stoned the train, the second time they stoned the bus, and the third time they were in a hurry and couldn't wait for the bus and so just stoned us while we waited for it. They liked their stones in Grimsby.

Turning back to my workplace, all this professorial absenteeism means the department is now run by Germans, Swedes and women. I wouldn't mind if it were Swedish women but by 'women' I mean the secretaries and a new woman called Morganna from Fleetwood, the town near Blackpool, not the pop group, Fleetwood Mac, who for some inexplicable reason reminds me of George Formby. Whenever I see her I start humming 'When I'm Cleaning Windows'. What with the Germans, annexing sociology, Morganna/George, the secretaries beginning to act more and more like the SS, and the excessive bureaucracy and memos telling us what we must do, the department is getting more and more like a WW2 Prisoner Of War camp every day. Nevertheless, after a bad start to the academic year, see below, I've been going in more to show I am still alive and available to collect my salary. I've discovered the building is very strange – you never see anyone. Sometimes I hear Morganna strumming on her ukulele two doors away; well, that's what it sounds like anyway. Mostly I only see my Korean PhD student, who lives outside my office and hasn't sobered up since his country unexpectedly reached the semi-finals of the World Cup.

There is also a man in the office opposite mine who for months I called Jim, but I recently discovered his name is Rab, and he is Scottish. He spends his evening re-enacting battles with toy soldiers and is, I believe, totally mad. He never goes home and constantly sees those undergraduate people who clutter the place up. I no longer teach undergraduates, only graduates, which I do prefer, although I will probably have to learn Chinese to be able to speak to them. I tutor graduates, notably the three Miss Lees who always arrive an hour or so early for meetings and sit outside my office chattering and giggling in Chinese, while they wait. Our meetings are very short. I ask them in English if everything is OK and they answer in Chinese. They do not appear to speak English and I have no idea what they are saying. There is then a great deal of giggling and bowing and they leave. I've thought of trying to talk to them in French or Spanish, which I could probably just about manage, but I doubt it would make any difference. It is all a total mystery to me.

But I digress. In truth, 2002 seems to have been a year in which we never had enough time to do things. So, what has been happening? It's no good hiding because I'm going to tell you whatever you do. The good news was the birth of our grandson on 19 April, Alan James weighed in at just over nine pounds. The bad news was the father disappearing after three weeks, although he has returned on a part-time basis, and so we've had to clear up the mess. As a result I've made lots of new friends: Mandy in the Council Offices, Jim in Housing Benefits, Mrs. Cartwright and Mrs. Whittaker in Income Support. I now realise the unemployed are not lazy; it's a full-time job chasing the benefits you're entitled to. We've also had to move Angie three times, an absolute nightmare! Fortunately, the father's mother and step-father have stayed on board, very much so, and help in all kinds of ways. In fact, they have become good friends. We had a christening in November and Alan is now a good Catholic boy.

So, big upheavals in Angie's life and also for Clare. She eventually got BCC for her 'A' Levels, but should definitely have got ACC, and probably ABC. She was a victim of the OCR 'A' Level cock-up and lost her first-choice university place, Bristol. Thankfully, BCC was what her second choice, Cardiff, wanted and so she went there to read Music. A month ago, the government claimed only 87 kids were affected, and the papers had it down to 24 last week. By next year it will probably never have happened at all and by the year after it will all be the fault of interfering parents and kids who deliberately chose to do worse than expected so that they could go to their second-choice university. Fortunately, Clare is quite happy, Cardiff is a decent university and she may well be better off there than Bristol. She's got superb accommodation, has made lots of friends, it's cheaper to live in Cardiff, there is a direct train to Worcester and the music department seems as good as Bristol's. It leans more towards those areas that particularly interest Clare. Oh, and on the proud parent front, I must add that Clare passed Grade 8 in both piano and flute this year, on the same day, with distinction in both cases. All's well that ends well.

Lizzie and James are doing fine. They both still go to Stagecoach but haven't appeared in anything. Lizzie is doing well at school, James a bit less so, his performance is very uneven. He struggles with maths but is above average in English. Lizzie has now definitely entered teenagerhood and we can do little except wait for her to re-emerge as a human being in a few years' time.

We have gained a rabbit from Angie - she can't keep pets where she is living now - but lost Cat Number Two, (daughter of Cat Number One). She just disappeared one night in late October. It doesn't entirely surprise me, I always thought she was a few chunks short of a can of Whiskas. She probably decided she was a tree and starved to death in a wood.

Anne continues to nurse but is increasingly overworked,

like all nurses, and spends much of her day driving around the hospital carpark looking for a space. One of the consultants nearly had his car clamped recently, apparently having to operate was not a good enough excuse.

I'm keeping my head above water. My efforts to keep going were not helped by having to miss the first two weeks of the new academic year in October. I went into hospital to have a hernia repaired. The operation was cancelled twice so it was quite frustrating, but the experience was much better than I thought it would be. It's quite restful being in hospital, although the nurses don't always help. The man in the next bed to me said to one nurse, "Why are you waking me up at 5.30 in the morning to take my blood pressure?" I thought it as very brave of him to say that as the night staff were male and looked like East German security guards. Come to think of it, he did disappear the following day. We have a brand-new hospital at Worcester, which is pretty neat. The problem is there are too many offices and not enough beds! But the beds they do have come with personal entertainment systems: radio, TV (15 channels), personal phone (I phoned Anne and my sister within an hour of coming around) and internet access, (not switched on). You have to pay a bit but it's fantastic, a bit of the future that does work.

Well, I suppose I'd better bring my ramblings on 2002 to a close. It's not been a very exciting year but there have been big changes, a grandchild and only two of the children are now living at home. But we'll all be here together for Christmas, pulling the crackers and reading out the old jokes, such as:

- Why did the elephant cross the road?
- Because it was tied to the chicken's leg.

James told me that one.

Have a peaceful and merry Christmas, and send your children to the University of Edgbaston.

DECEMBER 2003

Here we are again, another year been and gone, and another Christmas rapidly approaches. I'm hoping this Christmas is a bit better than last year, which was a bit dull. We had an even quieter New Year, babysitting our grandson overnight. I'm not very keen on babies, they are so small I'm always frightened I'm going to drop them, and having four of my own hasn't helped. I'm much happier with him now he's grown up a bit. He eventually had his first birthday in April, it took about a year, and by then he was much more fun. He's a very jolly little chap (he'll learn) and takes great delight in pursuing the cat at a high-speed crawl. I'm not sure which is funnier, the high-speed toddler or the even higher-speed cat. It's true to say that we had a much better night the day before New Year's Eve. It was Lizzie's 14th birthday, and we took her and ten of her friends on the Worcester Ghost Walk which was very entertaining with the effects much heightened by the reactions of 11 screaming teenage girls. To be honest, I thought the teenage girls were more frightening than the ghosts.

On the work front, I struggle on. I did manage a brief trip

to a small conference in the States in June. It was a fairly uneventful trip, apart from the crazy woman on the train to London. She suddenly stood up and asked us if we thought it fair they were serving caviar in first class. Fortunately, apart from one other man and me who studiously read our newspapers, there was only one family within earshot and they were even stranger than her, but in a quiet sort of way. Ms. Crazy was forced to march up and down the train muttering to herself, presumably everyone thought she was on a mobile phone, and so she eventually sat down, defeated. I seem to attract these people. I was sat on a bus on the way to the airport on my way home, behind two American ladies in their 50s when one turned to the other and said, "I must buy a telescope today, we're very close to Mars." I looked out of the window but I couldn't see it.

In my opinion, the worst thing about going to the States is getting into the country in the first place. You have to fill in this bizarre form to say you are not bringing any explosives, peanut butter sandwiches, camels or a sense of humour, and stand in line until a stony-faced immigration official stares at the form and your passport for a minimum of three minutes before letting you in. I queued for over an hour as the queue gradually got bigger. There are probably some people still there, desperately trying to calm an increasingly-restless camel, hidden in their hand luggage, by feeding it peanut butter sandwiches. I also object to standing in the non-US National line with all the other foreigners. There ought to be a special 'Non-US Nationals From Countries Whose Prime Minister Helps Us Bomb Other Countries Without Asking Too Many Questions (No French or Gypsies)' line. I don't even like the country all that much. Well, not so much dislike, as can never forgive a country that could produce Coca-Cola, the Osmonds and Ruby Wax. And potentially even less forgivable, is there a George Bush III out there?

Back in Blighty, the department continues to be run by a kind of female mafia. A sort of cross between the (select according to age) Mitford-Beverley-Nolan-Redmond sisters and Gestapo officers in drag, with senior academics as front men. It's a bit like having Sooty and Sweep in charge, I keep expecting the deputy head of department to start playing a trumpet, or produce a water pistol and squirt it at one of the secretaries.

No deviation from bureaucratic norms is allowed and it's only a matter of time before the principle of taking registers, even for graduate classes, is extended to staff, and our own families are only allowed to see us by appointment. Research is increasingly something we are supposed to produce in our own time, that is, during the night. I'd hate to be starting out now, many of the junior staff never seem to go home. Even if they get to the top of the greasy pole, the rewards are not comparable with other professions. Fortunately for me, there's nothing left for them to give me, except a decent-sized office and a nice pension. It's depressing , and academia is a dispiriting place to work these days. I'm hoping my son will do better than me and become an electrician perhaps, or even a plumber.

I was rather semi-detached in the department for much of the first half of the year, talking only to Mad Rab opposite, my PhD students, my head of the department, and the two other longest-serving members of the department. One is now semi-retired, although it's hard to tell what difference this makes; the other even more detached than me. My detachment is enhanced by the fact that I don't teach undergraduates any more. Most of the students think I'm an eccentric recluse, or I don't exist, while most of the staff regard me as a kind of mystery man who doesn't bring chocolates. I have toyed with the idea of playing the lunatic in the hope of being left completely alone, but so many academics wander around talking to themselves, looking dishevelled, and really are lunatics, I probably wouldn't get noticed.

Come to think of it, that's no longer true. Academia is getting more and more like snooker; faceless youngsters replacing the old characters. In my early days, we had people like Crazy Charlie, a Swedish Professor of Sociology who was completely unintelligible. God knows what group of misfits sat on the panel that appointed him, and apparently thought he would be able to give lectures. I can only imagine the other candidates were also swedes – of the vegetable variety –and Charlie got it on the arm and leg count. He was a dead ringer for the Swedish chef on the Muppets, and there used to be near-fistfights to avoid sitting next to him at Faculty Board.

Then there was Tim Dunne in my own department, our only professor for many years. Tim never wrote a lecture in his life. He just wrote books, on anything; the Jeffrey Archer of academia. There was another Tim Dunne in the university, a famous professor of history with an international reputation. There is a story that he was invited to address a big international conference in the States, only our Tim got the invitation by mistake and, without breaking sweat, popped over and did the job for him. I must confess I've always had a soft spot for Tim. He was very kind to me when I first started at the university, by which time he was already a professor, and I was even less significant than I am now. I inherited his office

– I was waiting outside with my desk the day he retired to make sure I got it first.

In a different world, Charlie and Tim would probably be selling the Big Issue at University station; everyone else is. Indeed, Tim would be writing it! On a related matter, bear with me, have you noticed how difficult it is to buy food at a supermarket these days? And how it gets even more difficult as Christmas approaches? First of all, you have to hand out large quantities of 20 pence pieces to random beggars. At the entrance to the supermarket you have to give to several charities and, of course, buy two to three copies of the Big Issue. Then you have to get some change to have a pound to insert into a trolley, having used the pound you had to buy a Big Issue. Hours later on the way out, you give most of your food away to those people with trolleys allegedly collecting tins of food for charity. Of course, as you take your pound out of the trolley you are immediately accosted by someone selling the Big Issue, and buy yet another one just to escape. Does anyone ever read that thing? It's become so much part of our daily lives I'm convinced sooner or later I shall go to the bathroom in the middle of the night, and there'll be a reformed burglar at the bathroom door who's broken in to sell me the Big Issue. I'd probably buy one!

Returning to the subject of work, things were going splendidly in September, until, on the first day of the new academic year, disaster struck. My foot had been playing me up for a while, and something happened on the way to the station - like I'd trodden on a red-hot poker. I got to the station and caught the train to Worcester but had to get a taxi home, and then spent two days literally crawling around the house. I couldn't put any weight on my right foot.

After various medical consultations, I ended up with my foot in plaster for two weeks. The fact that this happened on the first day of the Rugby World Cup was pure coincidence! Do you realise you can now get plastered in a choice of colours? Not just white but red, green, black, even purple. If you broke both arms and a leg you could have red, yellow and green and look like a set of traffic lights. I eventually decided I didn't want to make a fashion statement and would stick with white. I had a small broken bone in my right foot, and there was nothing much to be done except to wait for it to heal, and keep away from small hungry dogs. Apparently, my right foot has been worrying a lot lately and I have a stress fracture. However, things eventually got worse. I went back and they put on another plaster, which I still have on, and will do until the end of November. I was tempted to copy the man before me and have a Dennis the Menace (black and red stripes, I kid you not!) but eventually decided to stick with white again.

The year 2003 was quite a big one for us, we both reached 50 and had our silver wedding anniversary in August. We thought about having a party but in the end decided we'd rather be on holiday in our favourite place, the Scillies. There is a rather nice little Catholic church on the seafront. It is unusual because it is on the first floor in a block of terraced cottages, literally over the road from the sea. We went to 8 am Mass; it was a Tuesday and so there was just us, two professional Catholics and an ancient priest who sounded remarkably like Clement Freud and stumbled over his words. I had to stop myself from shouting out 'hesitation', and, of course, a load of boats bobbing around in the harbour outside the window.

We followed this with a slap-up breakfast in a restaurant

overlooking the sea, spent the day on our favourite island and went out in the evening to a tiny French restaurant, the sort where the chef comes around the tables at the end to ask questions. Rather a good day, and quite a good holiday overall, although the sea crossing on the way back was a bit rough. Anne and Lizzie love that, James has mixed feelings, but Clare and I both hate it, though we have different strategies to cope with it. I go to the bottom cabin and lie down with the sickies, plug myself into my music, pretend to be somewhere else and refuse to move until we dock. Clare follows the 'it's better if you can see the sea' school of thought, and sits on deck literally shaking with terror. We eventually got home at 5 pm on the Saturday and at 5.30 pm the electricity switched itself off. Fortunately, one of my daughters has had the good sense to include an electrician's daughter amongst her circle of friends, and so he came and sorted us out.

I suppose I'd better get around to talking about my family. Angie is now settled in a small but rather nice Council house about a mile away from us. Her relationship with Alan's father is mostly off rather than on, but his mother is very much still involved, although his step-father sadly died after a long spell in hospital this year.

Clare is now in her second year at Cardiff University, with a nice big room, I know because I put two coats of emulsion on the walls. The room is in a house shared with five friends, quite near the university, and she seems quite happy. Lizzie has started her GCSEs and James began secondary school in September. Both of them have been very busy rehearsing because they are in the pantomime Cinderella at a theatre in Warwick. It runs from 20th December to 3rd January, so you still have time to rush out and buy tickets.

Anne is still working at the new hospital and impersonating superwoman in her spare time, especially while I have my leg in plaster. Millie the cat has amazingly survived beyond her fourth birthday, having got over a minor traffic accident, and Starsky the rabbit, as I call him, think about it, 1970's American police TV series, keeps moving and so we keep feeding him and putting him in his run.

So here we are, Christmas on the way, and we'll be back to full strength in a couple of weeks when Clare returns. I hope you and yours are doing well and have a happy and peaceful Christmas and remember, if you are at a loose end this Christmas, there's an excellent pantomime on in Warwick, or failing that, a National One rugby match, Worcester versus Coventry, the day after Boxing Day.

Merry Christmas and a Happy New Year!

NOVEMBER 2004

Well, here we are, Christmas 2004. Actually, I still bear the scars of Christmas 2003, with all that driving to Warwick so the kids could appear in their pantomime. It was worth it though, and the kids' pantomime was rather better than the awful professional pantomime we saw on Boxing Day. The first half of this was dire, probably the worst hour I've spent since I inadvertently woke up in, stayed awake in, and listened to, one of my own lectures a few years ago. The script was terrible: whoever wrote it obviously thought that if he/she included every element of a pantomime, in no particular order, then it would be OK to do without a plot. It wasn't. The script was so thin it was positively anorexic. The only thing missing was a pantomime horse, though thinking about it, there probably was one at the beginning but it had the good sense to run away and join a circus, or give itself up to a French butcher. The good fairy with a 60 fag-a-day habit and a voice to match, Olive from the old sitcom 'On the Buses' was basically just there to draw her wages. Frankly, if she turned up and offered me three wishes, my first one would be for her to bugger off back to the bus depot, the second would be to stay there, and the third would be to hit my old biology teacher with a stick, for no particular reason except for a very old grudge and gratuitous violence. The two chaps from the Archers were totally redundant and should have stayed on the farm. The only good thing was the villain who was one of those actors that you see all the time on TV but can never remember their name. I'd tell you who he was but I can't remember his name. To be fair, the 'star', Nigel as was in 'EastEnders' if that means anything to you, did work really hard and at least got your sympathy by the end, but no-one could have rescued such a dreadful production.

I've seen a pantomime virtually every year now for 15 years at least, and I have to say I can count the good ones on the fingers of one hand. They are mostly mediocre, frequently poor and every so often absolutely dreadful. You get this mixture of ex-soap opera stars, often Australian, who can't tell jokes, comedians who can't get on television anymore, 'names', who for some reason were famous in the past but have now been forgotten, who can't do anything, kids in the chorus from the local drama school who can't stand or sit still, plus a man who likes dressing up as a woman or a farmyard animal. And who do we take to see this bunch of weirdos and has-beens? Why our children, of course! And, even if the acting were good, we all know the story and how it ends, the plots are always thin and pretty stupid. Have you ever thought about some of them, Dick Whittington, for example? That was the one we saw in Malvern. This guy really thinks London's streets are paved with gold, so what do they do with him when he gets there? Give him a nice comfy padded cell and call the psychiatric ward of a London hospital? No, they make him mayor, of course! Although, come to think of it, Ken Livingstone was elected mayor of London and so perhaps this is a bad example.

And then there is Cinderella. Are we seriously meant to believe she lives in a country where no-one else has the same shoe size as her? Come to think of it, this may also be a bad example as well. After many years of shopping with Anne, I have come to the conclusion she is a unique size in everything. But you know what I mean, the plots tend to make 'The Three Bears' look like a deep psychological thriller. And talking of that story, why are mummy and daddy bear in separate beds? Is their marriage on the rocks? Do we really feed this stuff to our pre-school kids? And what's this story about an old man with a white beard, who creeps into children's bedrooms late at night and gives them presents if they're good. The mind boggles! Eventually, we decided to give pantomimes and their dodgy plots a miss this year, oh no we didn't! Yes, we did, we're going to see Lord of the Rings III on Boxing Day.

But I digress, 2004 has, for me, been the year of the foot. Yes, I'm about to bore you with my operations! My broken foot, which those of you with long memories and amazing powers of staying awake may recollect, didn't mend properly despite six weeks in plaster towards the end of last year. I eventually had an operation in April to have a pin put in it. My hospital experience was slightly surreal, although perhaps it's just me noticing oddities as usual. I got into hospital at 8 am and in no time at all they had me stripped down for action with a big arrow written on my right foot. It is very important to be labelled correctly in hospital, Many years ago I shared a pre-surgery waiting room with three other men in Sheffield; two of us were in to have cysts removed, the other two were in for vasectomies. I made damn sure the arrow was in the right place, I can tell you.

They then kept me hanging around for two hours, just long enough for me to be operated on over, and so miss, lunch, the only hot meal of the day as this was the day unit where you are not supposed to stay overnight. I didn't feel too good afterwards and so I did stay overnight, as there were no beds on the wards. Unfortunately, there is no TV nor radio on the day unit, but luckily (!!!) I was in a windowless room with three men in their 80s, and so we talked. We did keeping pigeons, Llandudno (two of the men were Welsh), how I moved to Worcester from Welshpool in 1934 (a monologue in three parts, performed twice daily with additional performances when anyone new arrived), the contents of the Daily Mirror on both days, especially the six pictures of Lord Bath of Longleat, which led to a digression on local stately homes and toby jugs (don't even ask!), operations I have had and illnesses I may have, and probably more. I was losing the will to live by the end and rapidly becoming a supporter of euthanasia. I did perk up a bit when one of them said that after he got out of hospital the last time he felt like an 18year old, but when I asked him if he'd found one he didn't seem to understand the question.

I was eventually let out at 11.45 am and so just missed lunch again, the only cooked meal...

So, there I was, plastered to the knee for seven weeks and no weight to be put on my right foot. My only means of getting around was by hopping on my one good foot, while clinging on to a Zimmer frame. I am not joking, that last bit is really true. Worst of all, I wasn't able to bowl to James in the garden for weeks. I would have had to be the wicket-keeper, or perhaps even the wicket with the plaster on, God knows it's hard enough to get a game going even when I'm fit. We are already heavily dependent on my daughters finding boyfriends who like cricket, and have to tie the cat to a chair at silly mid-on to make up the numbers.

To make matters worse, it was eventually discovered that the pin they'd put in my foot had broken in half, and the break in the bone had not healed at all! They decided I needed the old pin replaced by a bigger and better one, which they duly did, in an operation the week before the start of term. So, there I was, the start of the academic year disrupted for the third year running, home again with a bright lime green plaster on my leg, a Red Cross wheelchair and a Zimmer frame. I had strict instructions from the consultant, delivered in a personal 90-second visit to my bedside, which is a sort of medical equivalent to seeing God on the way to Damascus, or in my case, Doncaster, to put absolutely no weight whatsoever on my right foot for the next six weeks.

As it happened, I was in good company as Stephen Gerrard's injury, a fracture of the fifth metatarsal, was exactly the same as mine, though on the other foot, and Beckham and Rooney have also broken metatarsals. Unfortunately, I am not a fit footballer in his 20s, and my powers of recovery are somewhat slower.

I did manage to get an overnight stay on a ward this time, which meant I had access to a personal TV and phone. I was once again plagued by the over-80s, Bill and Ben as I called them, they were really called Paul and Randolph – I didn't make that up – but were quite literally unintelligible, just like Bill and Ben. They also waved to each other, one was opposite me and the other next to me, and quite possibly lived in flowerpots. They slept all evening and then about 1am Ben/Paul started shouting incoherently, except for the word 'light' – a bit like Father Jack shouts 'drink' in the 'Father Ted' series. This lasted for about three to four minutes, and was repeated at 15-minute intervals until 5.30. Bill/Randolph was less vocal, spilling drinks and unpicking his stitches were his specialities, but he did quite frequent 'hello, theres' in a high-pitched voice, a sort of cross between a castrated Val Doonican (now there's a pleasing thought - I remember his shows, fun for all the family, well, at least for his family) and a parrot with a serious drug problem.

Of course, the end result was that just as I was falling asleep, I was woken up again. I must admit I did have to laugh out loud at 3 am, although I could have killed them, which had the beneficial side-effect of one of the nurses making me a milky drink. Beneficial at a price because I think it may also have prompted her to write 'loony' in my notes. I took refuge in some tedious Brazilian and Dutch football on the TV, but even 180 minutes of that, with a total of only one goal, could not send me to sleep. I eventually got to sleep at 5.30 am by blocking them out with acoustic music on my Walkman, only to be woken up by a nurse to take my blood pressure at 6.30 am. Still, I felt pretty good and mostly enjoy being in hospital. In an odd sort of way it is rather relaxing, you can watch a lot of sport and get a lot of reading done without having to break off to drive a daughter somewhere.

After seven weeks, I switched to a walking plaster for a further three weeks, as the break in the bone appeared to be healing. I'm due to be completely plaster free at the beginning of December, and will be able to DRIVE again! I have been going to work one day a week, usually driven by Anne, and have done my teaching in a wheelchair. I think going to work once a week has probably kept me sane, although you may think otherwise after reading this letter. The upshot of all this is I've nothing much to report on the work front as I've not really been there very often.

Anne continues to work as a part-time nurse with a parking problem. Angie and Alan are fine. Angie still has her moments but is coping well and, although there seems little chance of them getting back together, the father of her child sees his son regularly, drives Angie to Tesco once a week, and was even on hand to light the fireworks in our garden this year. I couldn't, well, I could, but I couldn't get away from them fast enough. Clare is now, unbelievably, in her final year reading music at Cardiff. She seems to be enjoying herself tremendously this year, more playing and composition, and less writing of essays. Lizzie is doing her GCSEs and James is doing, well, as little as he can get away with. He's not 13 yet and already his voice has broken and he's taller than his mother.

So, all-in-all, 2004 has been a fairly quiet and slightly difficult year. Nevertheless, we approach Christmas in our usual state of panic, completely unprepared but looking forward to having all four of the kids, plus grandson, under the same roof for a few days. Christmas Day is one of those days when having four kids seems worth all the effort. I hope you and yours are well and I look forward to the day when our children will be old enough and rich enough to buy us a drink at Christmas, I've pencilled in 2016 for mine!!

Merry Christmas

P.S. Sadly, neither the rabbit with no name nor Millie the cat will be celebrating Christmas with us this year.

NOVEMBER 2005

Well, another year goes by and Christmas 2005 draws rapidly closer. We're trying to simplify things a bit this year. After last year we decided we were still treating our offspring like children and some of the longstanding family Christmas rituals needed to be jettisoned. In short it was time to have a more-adult orientated festive season. The kids will probably think this means they can go out more, get drunk and stay in bed until lunchtime, but Anne and I are interpreting this as meaning we don't have to do all the shopping and work, and we shall go out more, get drunk and stay in bed until lunchtime. I shall still have my wrestle with a real Christmas tree though, but we're dispensing with Christmas stockings for the kids, we may well go to Midnight Mass instead of going to church on Christmas morning, and watching 'The Snowman' on Christmas Eve and attendance at a pantomime on Boxing Day will cease to be mandatory. However, the children will all have to start eating sprouts and will have to learn how to operate the dishwasher. They will be told it is not the 'kitchen fairies' but their semi-drunken father, listening to his new Jethro Tull CD, who clears up the kitchen while they watch a film on Christmas afternoon, after their mother has collapsed from exhaustion.

So, what of 2005? Well, I was back into driving to the theatre at Warwick in March. Lizzie and James were in a surprise birthday show for the principal of their drama school, who is called Pat, and was, I don't know, probably 60 or 65. She runs the Worcester and Stratford Stagecoach franchises and does a great job, although she does tend to talk incessantly. I call it the Pat Rap. Her son is just as bad. He is very talkative but makes up for it by being an excellent performer. He really ought to have been spotted and become a children's TV presenter. He teaches the kids acting and stagecraft and, last Christmas, he told an incredibly convoluted story about how he knew Anthony Newley and, until he died, he and Pat used to receive a home-made Christmas card from Newley. If his card-making was anything like his singing, I'd have sent it back to him and told him not to be such a mean bugger. He should send a card with a badly-drawn picture of a Victorian horse and trap covered in snow from the bottom of a Woollies 50 for £2 box, like the rest of us. And let's face it, if you're going to name drop, you might as well pick someone who throws his money about and everyone has heard of. Who the hell remembers Anthony Newley? I suppose there must be some people out there who would say 'Isn't he that tight sod who wouldn't buy proper Christmas cards?' but probably no-one will remember him other than me. Me and the 43 others who bought 'Do You Mind' in 1959, I was only 6 years old at the time and heavily into Cliff Richard. I still play 'The Day I

Met Marie' very loudly in the car occasionally to Anne's great embarrassment, but I don't know the excuses of the other 42. On second thoughts, Mrs. Newley will certainly remember him, albeit mainly because she's still annoyed about the home-made birthday cards he used to send her.

If Pat's son wants to see someone famous, he ought to travel not act. I've seen Thora Hird and Arthur Scargill on Doncaster station. Unfortunately not together, what a News of the World story that would have made. Indeed, they might have been a good combination, Arthur could have given fiery sermons on Songs of Praise and Thora could have sold those chairlift things that go up and down stairs, the ones she's always advertising, to miners as a less stressful way of going down a pit. I've also seen Alan Whicker on an airport bus between terminals at Charles de Gaulle airport (where else!), and Harold Wilson buying pipe tobacco in the Scilly Isles.

Returning to the run up to Christmas, the driving to Warwick restarted in September as Lizzie and James are once again in the pantomime. It's easier this time because we know what to expect and how best to pass the time spent waiting for them to finish. I have to say, the whole thing makes me feel very Christmassy and Warwick has got some excellent pubs and restaurants. Anne did most of the early driving and I took over at the end of October. They're doing Snow White this year, which rules James out of consideration for a leading role (see below).

For once, we made some inroads into the house in 2005. The living room has been completely redone and Anne has finally got her much-desired polished wooden floor. We've also thrown a lot of things away. It's amazing what you accumulate and what you keep because you thought it might be 'useful' or it's 'interesting'. Why on earth did I keep a single drumstick used by Mott the Hoople's drummer at Doncaster Top Rank in 1970 for 35 years? Mind you, I also have a Doncaster Rovers versus Manchester United football programme dated 21 April 1945, which must be worth something.

Back to the house, my in-laws continue to visit and help. Anne's father still does bits. Quite big bits actually, considering he's turned 80, but my mother-in-law does rather less these days. She mainly irons, watches TV and rearranges things in the kitchen cupboards, although I suppose that's better than cupboarding, watching the iron and rearranging things inside the TV. I usually take the opportunity to spend more time in Edgbaston when they are around.

However, I remain fairly invisible at work. I knew a similar academic at Warwick when I was a PhD student. He kept his door locked much of the time, a trick I borrow when I'm busy. Unfortunately, he didn't quite have the knack of staying hidden because he used to wear an orange shirt with a green tie. It was so bright you could see him for miles. He used to cause chaos at traffic lights because everyone thought the lights were on amber and either tried to get through quickly or slammed on the brakes. He wrote about welfare economics and was, I think, the man who calculated the economic loss due to people being run over by cars, and came up with a negative value for women – mainly because he didn't allow for the contribution of non-working wives busy bringing up families and ironing orange shirts for their husbands. However, the logical conclusion of this was that it was economically advantageous to run women over. Had it been reported in the Daily Mail, thousands of women could have died. Fortunately, it only got as far as an academic journal and so, apart from a few rogue economists in university towns, hanging around traffic lights in orange shirts and fast cars looking for women pedestrians, and the editors of unreadable economic journals like 'Econometrica' having to be rounded up, this particularly brainless contribution to economic research had little impact. However, it was one of the reasons I decided I wanted to live in the real world, and work in an interdisciplinary department rather than be an academic economist. Being an academic is unreal enough for me. But there are worse journals than 'Econometrica'. I came across one at a conference called the 'Journal of Holocaust Studies'. Can you imagine that landing on your mat every three months? What a jolly read that must be.

In any case, I need to go to work more often as I'm trying to re-establish myself there a bit. We're still appointing lots of new people and it's getting harder and harder to keep up. Frankly, they look so young I can't tell them apart from the PhD students, we have about 40 of those, or visiting policemen – they are getting younger as well.

I still wander around the department smiling benignly at everyone, but I've developed my act and now probably sound increasingly like the Queen, as I say things like "And what do you do?" "Is that difficult?" "Do you like corgis, as well? and "If Phillip does that again, tell him to give the melon back, put his trousers on and wait for me in the car." It seems to work most of the time, although I did spend 20 minutes talking about American foreign policy to a cleaning lady, before she asked me to lift my feet up so she could vacuum under my desk, and I realised she wasn't our new lecturer in international relations after all.

Many of the people at work continue to think I don't exist or I'm some sort of mystery man. A spy perhaps, or an undercover university security man. Actually, our security men are not so much undercover as under siege. Theft is rampant on the campus. Even the security men are potential victims. I remember working late one evening when we first moved into our new building a couple of years ago, and a security man coming into my office and asking who I was and when I was leaving. Checking up, you think? Not exactly, he was popping out before coming back to do the nightshift ,and wanted somewhere safe to leave his portable TV so he could watch the football later on. I did rather well and got £40 for it.

The beginning of the academic year 2005/06 has been my best for years. I'm not in hospital, in plaster, in a wheelchair or in a drunken stupor, and I seem to be on top of things and reasonably well-prepared for my teaching for the first time this century. I appear to have inherited an additional half-course, which means I'm teaching something I don't know too much about, well, not in detail, but this has never held me back before. Students tend to be fairly gullible and sheep-like, and provided they get good lecture notes they don't really care much what you tell them, as long as you sound authoritative and include the occasional joke.

Funnily enough, students haven't changed much, even though they now pay more money in fees. I suspect they will not change much, at least at first when it gets really expensive, as it will from next year. Choosing a university will become much more like going to the supermarket with cut price deals and special offers. Places like Edgbaston will mostly charge full fees, but some of the newer universities that were formerly colleges, like Luton, Derby and Worcester, may well become like that furniture shop with near-permanent sales. Digressing briefly, do you ever think somewhere out there is a man who paid full-price for his MFI furniture? What an idiot!

I feel sorry for undergraduates today. In my day, we not only didn't have to pay any fees, but actually received a means-tested grant. I received nearly the full grant, to which I was able to add a small contribution from my parents. I managed well enough on this and was able to do without a parental contribution when I began to receive a slightly larger postgraduate grant, and thus achieved financial independence. Today's students receive nothing and have to take out loans to pay fees and living costs, and leave university with the three Ds – degree, debt and depression. They are hit by a triple whammy when they leave university because they not only have their student debt to pay off, but also want to buy a house and provide for a pension. They don't stand a chance. I think if the present system was in operation when I was 18, I would not have gone to university.

Returning to how to behave as an academic, I still think occasionally about going all the way and playing the mad professor. It's been done before and better and, as I've said in previous letters, eccentric academics are a dying breed – it's all efficiency and money. But we still get the odd one thankfully. We still have Mike, a former head of department who is not so much eccentric as loud and larger than life, with a tendency to get drunk on social occasions, and whenever he goes shopping for clothes. The only other one in my department is Mad Rab in the office opposite to mine, who I've mentioned before. It's hard to say much about him because he is Scottish, and therefore largely unintelligible. He supports football teams with strange names, like Inverness Thistle and Ross County, which sound like characters in a glossy American soap opera. He spends too much time with students, and wanders into my office with silly quotes from students' exam papers and essays. You know the sort of thing, students who think Karl Marx was the younger brother of Groucho, Chico and Harpo but couldn't act and so became a shopkeeper who joined forces with Earl Spencer and created M&S.

Some of the misunderstandings are truly very funny, although some gaps in undergraduates' knowledge are staggering, not to say frightening. Personally, I long since gave up on students, and indeed younger academics. However, I prefer the company of people who can remember Herman's Hermits, hum the theme tune of 'Z-Cars' and name at least one member of Black Sabbath or Deep Purple - Ozzy Osbourne does not count. The other members of Black Sabbath were Toni Iommi and Geezer Butler – I can't remember the name of the drummer and, for Deep Purple, Ian Gillan (vocals),Ian Paice (drums), Ritchie Blackmore (guitar), Roger Glover (bass) and Jon Lord (keyboards). If they can also remember 'Torchie the Battery Boy' and know Cliff Richard's real name (Harry Webb), I'll buy the drinks. And, if they know the title of the first ever episode of 'Dr. Who' (`An Unearthly Child') and can remember who was the star of 'The Avengers' before John Steed/Patrick MacNee joined the programme then I'll buy dinner as well. (The original lead was Ian Hendry. I believe he was avenging something at the very beginning - his wife's murder, I think.)

However, I do know Rab still spends all his spare time wearing an anorak and making model soldiers, and then fighting battles with them, in which the Scottish always beat the English. He is mostly harmless, except of course when drunk from January 1st to 4th each year. He does cycle to and from work though, and takes his bike up to his office in the lift. I always find that disturbing. It seems to me that anyone who needs to take a bicycle with them in the lift on the way to their office, either completely lacks confidence and/or conversational skills, or has a bizarre sense of what is really valuable. If we all did it, it would get ridiculous, lecture theatres full of bicycles, people fixing punctures in the corridors. And why stop at bicycles? Why not back the Volvo into the lift and take that to your office as well? With a bit of luck you might crush a few of those bloody bicycles! I could understand if Rab used the bicycle in lectures, as giving lectures from a bicycle has a certain appeal and could be very stylish. You could do a wheelie to emphasise a point, and could make a great entrance by riding down the stairs from the top of the lecture theatre. Another thing I've always fancied is giving a lecture on stilts.

The other occupant of morning lifts I find disturbing is the sweaty jogger. They are usually a closet marathon runner, and often disappear altogether after a few years, having been knocked over by a milk float while running in the dark at 5 am. Or transform themselves in later years into a shambolic wreck, barely able to walk, their knees damaged beyond repair by the constant pounding they received in their jogging days. They also have a tendency to hurl themselves violently to one side whenever anyone shouts "Milk float". Ultimately though, it's probably not a good career move to become a mad academic, although being a milkman has a certain appeal.

So, I struggle on. We've just appointed a Japanese

academic as head of department, as all the other professors have either just done it, or are ill (me), are drunk and running another department, sulking in Southeast Asia, running their own alternative department/empire, or have got a better job at another university. Personally, I wouldn't want to be head of department if they offered me all the furniture in MFI, even if it were pre-assembled for me. It was very different in the old days, of course, when being head of department only meant you had to stay awake until the end of departmental meetings, and remember to switch the light out and shut the door on the way out. But now it's a treadmill and everything has to change all the time. It's like being in a permanent Cultural Revolution. The most recent and craziest example is that having moved out of a dilapidated 1960s tower block, served by completely inadequate lifts, to a brand new, purpose-built building four years ago, they are now talking about moving back to the tower. Does no-one have a memory here? The only department that chose to stay in the building was Social Policy, and they only did it because they train social workers, and working in a semi-derelict tower block is part of their training. Still, with so many German lecturers in the department at least meetings and lectures should start on time. Nowadays, we have a lot of non-Brits in our department and our staff profile is beginning to look like the team sheet of an 'English' football team. I've got fed up with office politics and retreated back into the pleasures of my youth. I've started reading non-academic stuff again, mostly modern novels and some old favourites like George Orwell.

I suppose I'd better say something about the family. James has become a teenager and is rapidly approaching 6ft tall, 5ft 9ins on his 13th birthday, and probably eating and/or listening to loud music as I write. Hence his unsuitability for a leading role in 'Snow White and the Seven Dwarves' referred to earlier in this letter. He managed to get himself suspended from school for three days in March, which is a bit like punishing a child for stealing sweets by forcing them to eat chocolate. His offence was letting off stink bombs in the school corridor. We had to go to a 'reintegration meeting' with his head of year, who turned out to be Welsh, thirty-ish and dressed in shorts. I presume he was a PE teacher or had just got out of bed. Come to think of it, I sincerely hope he was a PE teacher. When Anne questioned the sense of James missing three days' schooling, he said, (you have to imagine a man in shorts, with a heavy Welsh accent at this point), "Well, Mrs Redmond, we 'ad to do something. The 'ole school stank for days!" We laughed all the way back to the car. It's reassuring to know that men in shorts are patrolling our school corridors with deodorant sprays set on 'kill'.

Going back to loud music, to their horror, and I suspect I am not alone in this, I quite like most of the music my youngest two children play. Thinking about it, I am probably doing them terrible psychological damage by asking them to turn it up rather than down when I go into the room. I do, however, stand firm in my dislike of rap, and anything involving steel drums or Cilla Black.

Clare completed her degree at Cardiff and got a 2:1. We went down for the ceremony, in that very hot spell in mid-July. To be completely accurate, it was unbearably hot. We stayed over the night before but hardly slept in the heat. Normally I avoid these ceremonies like the plague but I couldn't get out of this one. It was strangely nostalgic as I graduated there myself thirty years earlier, virtually to the day. Clare is now hoping to do a Master's degree in performance and is preparing for the auditions.

Lizzie was also on the exam trail. She passed all her GCSEs with approximately a three-way split between As, Bs and Cs. She also managed to get her picture in the local paper twice this year. The first time was her arrival at the school leavers' ball. The kids turned up in all manner of vehicles, including an ambulance. "All we need now is a fire engine," said one of the teachers, and Lizzie and six friends arrived in a fire engine. The second time was when she had the dubious honour of playing for, and meeting, Mrs. Thatcher at her music school. She has now started 'A' Levels and acquired a boyfriend.

Angie and Alan are doing quite well, no disasters this year so far, and Alan has started pre-school nursery, or whatever they call it. Alan's father has had a less-good year having become prone to drunken driving. I spent a jolly Boxing Night or, to be precise 3 am to 4am on 27 December, waiting outside the police station to collect him. It's still hard to dislike him though - possibly less so in the middle of the night; he just needs to grow up a bit, that's all.

That's it, another year come and gone. The Parkinson's is a bit worse but I still manage to work, at a reduced pace, drive and function fairly normally, although I can see early retirement getting rather nearer. We seem to have stopped going to the Young Parkinson's Group. We never had much in common with them except for the disease, and I quickly became the only one still working and one of the few with kids still at school. I also find it's all a bit too institutionalised for me. And at this time of year, there is always the threat that Jim (see previous letter) will turn up with his guitar, or violin, or whatever, and start playing 'God Rest Ye Merry Gentlemen' very badly and we'll be expected to join in. It wouldn't be so bad if he'd play something appropriate like 'Shaking All Over'. My God, it just occurred to me. Jim may have even formed a band, which is a terrifying thought to end the letter with.

Have a good Christmas.

DECEMBER 2006

Here we are again, another year, another letter from that lunatic in Worcester. The year began with the tail end of the pantomime at Warwick, and this was followed by exhaustion. Noel Coward was right: "Don't put your children on the stage, Mrs. Worthington." Christmas 2005 was a slightly less childlike Christmas as planned, although Anne did rather undermine the decision to abandon stockings, by wrapping and putting what would have gone in the kids' stockings in gift bags under the Christmas tree. We managed to acquire three real Christmas trees, admittedly one was a two-foot freebie, which was probably over the top. On the other hand, for the first time for years, we had quite a relaxed Christmas Eve and did not spend the day frantically trying to finish everything. I'm not sure what we did right but I hope to repeat it this year.

The big news of the year is that we have another grandchild, a granddaughter, courtesy of Angie – with a different father. We would prefer her to stay by herself as neither of the fathers of her children seem to be entirely suitable for her. They're not bad people and are still around a great deal, but we have come to the conclusion they are probably not always a good influence on our grandchildren. The new addition is called Dallas. It could have been worse, Angie could have insisted on Minneapolis, or Little Rock, or even Salt Lake City. Dallas is a proper name (I looked it up), and it means 'living on a clearing'. No, I'm none the wiser either. It is also more widely used as a boy's name, which further adds to the confusion. Angie is doing OK and is fiercely independent, although she does need some help from time to time. I'm sure there will be many crises to come but, I'm rather proud of her in many ways. Nothing has been easy for her.

After a year at home and a complicated life involving three part-time jobs, four if you include giving piano lessons in the evening, Clare has now returned to Cardiff. She's at the Royal Welsh College of Music and Drama, not the University, to do a two-year Masters in Music (Performance). She seems to be having a marvellous time and enjoying being a graduate much more than she did an undergraduate. The longstanding boyfriend is now merely a 'friend' and she is a free agent.

Lizzie is still with her boyfriend, of whom we continue to approve. She will complete her 'A' Levels in the summer of 2007 and hopefully go on to university. James has just begun his GCSEs and we await his progress as much in hope as in expectation as he is not very enthusiastic about school, to put it mildly. Anne continues to work but with an ever-growing hatred of getting up at 6.15 am to do an 'early', and ever-growing despair about the state of the National Health Service in general, and the car park at Worcester Royal Infirmary in particular.

I too continue to work. It's becoming an increasingly weird

experience as the people I know leave or retire, to be replaced by new people whom I don't know. I am hoping I will eventually become invisible and they will continue to pay my salary without my having the bother of going in. My teaching has been changed again and is now completely different to what it was three years ago. I'm even teaching half a politics course, which is a bit strange as I don't even have an 'A' Level in Politics. I also remember specific assurances being given to the non-political science members of International Studies, that they would not be required to teach politics courses after we amalgamated in 1983.

Having said that, teaching something I know little about has never been a problem before. Students will write down anything you say and believe virtually anything you tell them. In any case, increasingly most of them are Chinese and don't even understand English. Moreover, since I was condemned as a fire hazard, I spend most of my time tidying up my office rather than teaching. It's amazing how much irrelevant material you gather in your office over 30 years. I added a real cracker of a book to my 'unsold and unsolicited books received' shelf this year. It was all about homosexuality in the European Union and included a chapter entitled 'Coming out of the closet in Slovenia'. The mind boggles! I didn't know they had closets, let alone homosexuals, in Slovenia. I'm now trying to work out how I can include it in one of my courses.

It seems to me that the department is going downhill at a rapid rate. Our best professor, one of my best friends in the department, together with the best of our younger academics, who the powers that be won't promote because he's too young, are all going to our arch-rivals, Warwick. Others seem set to follow. Our current head of department is totally out of his depth and has just about alienated everyone in the department. Those who can get away have done so. For example, two of our professors are currently hiding/sulking in Hong Kong and Australia, respectively. He's tried to push me into early retirement, which I've resisted strongly. I don't want to go just yet.

Our graduate school is in steep decline with only 70 students this year, compared to over 100 for each of the last three. Our head of department's response has been to avoid taking any decisions, by referring everything to a sub-committee, petulantly decree that no departmental money is to be spent on leaving dos for staff (especially the three going to Warwick), and to threaten to invade Poland with his German allies. Alright I made the last bit up, but he's definitely got his eye on France. It's all rather sad really, even Mad Rab in the office opposite to mine is depressed, I think it's driving him sane. He just sits there reading his books about Red Indians (don't ask) and muttering unintelligibly to himself in his thick Scottish accent. I think he is pining for the Scottish glens, will put on his kilt and head north soon, and probably be found wandering around Nuneaton – he has little sense of direction – looking for undergraduates.

Moving on to happier things, we seem to have spent much of the year attending weddings, two in one weekend in May, each quite different but both very enjoyable. The main thing they had in common was men in kilts (my letter has a Scottish flavour this year): a few real Scotsman and a couple of English impersonators at one wedding, and a Welshman at the other. What is it in the British male that makes him want to wear skirts? It always amazes me how men seem to lose no opportunity to dress up as women. You see it at rugby club parties all the time, great big hairy front row forwards with wigs and stockings on. We went to the Rocky Horror Show this year, all those men in tights doing the Time Warp. No, chaps, you don't look good, the words that come to mind are saddo, pillock, and ridiculous. There's no wonder we can't win the World Cup, the players are probably too concerned with not ruining their make-up or laddering their tights.

The second thing the two weddings had in common was excellent speeches. The best man at one of them would make a very good stand-up comedian. His comic timing was perfect, his style very Les Dawson-esque and, thank goodness, he wore trousers throughout. The third common factor was that at both weddings the groom went on stage during the evening entertainment and sang quite well. We also went to another good wedding in Wales in September. Fortunately this was kilt-less and the groom didn't sing although, being Welsh, he probably could have done if he'd wanted to. The bride was the daughter of an old friend of Anne's, whose ex-husband hails from Goole, only ten miles from my birthplace. I once saw some graffiti on a wall in Goole which said 'Goole is the arsehole of the world' and I think that was about right, possibly a bit unfair on arseholes. It was a minor river-port, and so the Germans bombed it during the war – allegedly. Personally, I think Hitler visited Goole in his youth and couldn't bear the thought of conquering a country with a town like Goole in it, and so tried to obliterate it before he sent his army in. The consequent delay probably made an important contribution to our winning the war.

Goole has featured significantly in my life twice. In 1957, when was four I spent my first and, until I was nearly 50, only night in a hospital there (as a patient, rather than as an unofficial visitor to the nurses' home, that is). I was there to have my adenoids out (in Goole Hospital). As far as I know, they are still there, presumably forlornly waiting to be transplanted into someone leaving the town. I have two memories of my stay in hospital. First, my bed had the only radio on the ward that did not work and, second, I hated the food. Both of these were important considerations for a 4 year old and so, on balance, I didn't like it there. In 1976 I failed my driving test for the second time in Goole. It was a strange place for a driving test, very flat and with only one main road, but what a road. It had a six-exit roundabout at one end, a T-junction at the other and in between every hazard you could think of. A pelican crossing, a zebra crossing, two giraffes and an elephant crossing, a railway crossing with a complicated multi-lane approach, if you got in the wrong lane you'd had it, and at least two sets of traffic lights. For all I knew, there were probably also wild deer, stray sheep and falling rocks, and the road was used as an emergency landing runway for airplanes during bad weather. If you could negotiate this road, you could drive anywhere. Consequently, the driving test consisted of driving up and down it twice before driving off in search of a hill on which to do a hill start. I failed because I made a mess of the roundabout, but I've never held it against the town or its inhabitants. Good grief, they suffer enough just opening the curtains every morning. No, I don't dislike the place but I wouldn't go there for a holiday, or another driving test.

Talking of holidays, we also travelled a bit in 2006. Unusually, Anne and I spent a few days in Brussels in July. I took her there nearly 20 years ago with a small party of students. The students insisted on staying in the cheapest hotel in town, I kept getting lost as it was only my second visit to

Brussels, it was cold and rained all the time, we spent all our time in anonymous EU buildings, Anne ate something that disagreed with her, and on the way home started to have a miscarriage. For some reason, Anne doesn't have good memories of her visit and so I've always felt I owed her a nice weekend in Brussels. This year we finally made it. Good weather, my favourite hotel the Metropole – the oldest hotel in Brussels if you ever go there, a great day in Bruges and they even put a pageant on in the Grande Place for us on the first evening. A few men waving flags about as my deeply unimpressed wife put it. To be fair, they did have horses as well. Thinking about it, it would have been a lot more exciting if they'd sat on the flags and waved the horses about.

We also managed a weekend in Paris, this time with Clare, Lizzie and James in tow. We stayed in a small hotel which, much to the amusement of the three kids, put them in what was virtually a suite and Anne and I in an extended broom cupboard. Incidentally, if you ever go to the Eiffel Tower, be sure to take three meals, a mobile toilet, a sleeping bag and a tent – you queue forever. The best bit of the visit was probably going to the top of the Arc de Triomphe. The children were not too taken by the Louvre, it does involve a lot of walking and gets so crowded, and all those photographers and video makers! I have now appeared in so many Japanese holiday videos I'm probably regarded as a minor film star in Japan!

Anne, James and I also spent two weeks in the Scillies in August, with Lizzie and Clare joining us for the last ten days. Amazingly, Anne, emboldened by her trips under the sea on Eurostar, after only a little persuasion agreed to go via the 20-minute helicopter ride rather than on the tedious, and often bumpy, two and three-quarter hour ferry trip. It was very noisy, but I have to admit my first words on landing were, "I'm never setting foot on that damn boat again." While the weather deteriorated on the mainland toward the end of August, it didn't on the Scillies (except for two days). Every day started cloudy but with sunshine breaking through by early afternoon at the latest, and very little rain. Our rented house was central and we had a marvellous time. For the first time ever, we walked all the way around the main island, over the course of three days, and discovered a small beach we didn't know existed. We had it all to ourselves for most of the afternoon. We also managed to visit all five of the smaller islands, even the tiny (a mile by half a mile) uninhabited one, Samson.

As Christmas approaches I find myself once more on the road to Warwick every Sunday, as James rehearses to appear in 'Aladdin'. Lizzie has temporarily retired from the stage in the face of 'A' Levels, but is finding time to play piano in her college's production of 'The Beggar's Opera' in December. At least I'm travelling in some style now, having dispatched the faithful, 12 year old Spacewagon via eBay. I've bought, or rather effectively leased, our first ever brand new Volkswagen Touran, which is a truly wonderful vehicle. I'm still driving in spite of the PD, although as I approach the end of my 11th year since being diagnosed, I must admit driving and work are getting harder. Some of the lack of energy is just due to getting older and it's all too easy to attribute every ache and pain to PD. It's best just to get on with it, as the Bishop said to the actress. I certainly hope to work for a few more years yet, and write a few more Christmas letters!

Well, that's it. Another year come and gone, the family will all be here on Christmas Day so it's almost time for my annual struggle with a Christmas tree, which will be taller than me. I always think there is something totally crazy about putting a (just about) live tree in the hall. I mean, why stop at a tree? Why not put a lawn down, a fishpond in the bathroom and grow a hedge in front of the bay window to replace the curtain? In truth, most of these Christmas traditions are relatively new and 150 years ago Christmas was quite different. And if Queen Victoria had not married Albert we would have quite different traditions (and Victoria would have got more sleep!). It all seems so random really, and yet the pressure to conform and behave as if Christmas has been like it is now for centuries, is overwhelming. My kids would be very unhappy if we didn't follow the usual routine, and even I get withdrawal symptoms if I don't sing 'O Little Town of Bethlehem' at least once over Christmas. I particularly like the lines: 'Yet in thy dark streets shineth, The everlasting light…'

Let's hope the everlasting light shines in both our streets this Christmas.

Merry Christmas and a Happy New Year!

DECEMBER 2007

It's nearly that time of year again. It hardly seems a few months since we struggled through last year's Christmas. It was not one of our more successful efforts, as we were exhausted from our almost daily trips to Warwick to take James to his damn pantomime. In addition, we took a crazy decision to buy a large piece of furniture, that required major re-organisation in the downstairs rooms of the house a couple of days before Christmas. The Christmas tree lights failed on Boxing Day and refused to light thereafter, despite my changing of fuses and much twiddling and tightening of bulbs. And the table collapsed towards the end of Christmas dinner, thankfully we'd just about finished and Lizzie grabbed the only remaining bottle of red wine as it went past her, and so the only serious casualty was half a glass of cider. In any case, the table has collapsed before and everyone seemed to enjoy the occasion well enough. Christmas, that is, not the table collapsing, and the kids even did much of the washing up, and so it didn't really matter.

I must begin by apologising for last year's Christmas letter, which reads far too much like a Christmas letter, a proper one! You will be relieved to know that in order to prevent repetition of the decline in standards, I intend to refer to family members and family news as little as possible this year. So, what of 2007?

Well, it was certainly a good (bad?) year for weather. To start with, we got heavy snow for a day in January. Bizarrely, Worcester was hardest hit in the entire country. Bizarre because it never snows here. We do floods (see below) and heat waves. The BBC weather station at Barbourne in north Worcester occasionally records the highest temperature of the day in the country, but not snow – only three times in the 20 years I've lived here. Of course, the day it snowed, every school in Worcestershire closed, there was gridlock in Edgbaston and one woman was featured on local radio because it took her nearly eight hours to drive from Hereford to Worcester, a journey of 23 miles. Mind you, it can take four hours in the summer if you get stuck behind a tractor, up to five if the farmer has been on the cider and keeps stopping to relieve himself.

A bit of snow and the UK grinds to a halt. God help us if we were ever hit by a tsunami. That's not strictly true everywhere. Where I'm from in South Yorkshire, the men just put on a tee-shirt and wade through the snow to the pub as if it were a normal day, leaving their wives to clear the snow off the drive and cook their dinner.

To be honest, that's not completely correct either. I did know a man who was an exception to this. I used to have a neighbour, a northerner, who would always clear his drive before he went to work. In fact, I think he used to be out during the night catching the snow in a bucket. He was universally hated by all the men for miles around for setting such a bad example and causing identical comments by all nearby wives at the breakfast table: "I see so & so has cleared his drive already. When are you going to do ours, then?" The smug sod used to wash his car and mow the lawn every Sunday in the summer as well, instead of going to the pub and reading the paper like the rest of us. He probably also did the shopping, cooking and ironing and didn't like sport either but preferred dressmaking and vacuuming the stairs. There's always one who spoils it for the rest. I like to think he ended up tripping over his own rake and suffocating in a huge pile of leaves he'd just raked up. Or possibly getting run over while clearing litter off the road outside his house, by one of his male neighbours probably. But in reality, as you read this, he's almost certainly still alive, polishing the tiles on his roof, with his extra-large (reindeer-size) pooper scooper at his side and laying down some plastic for the sleigh to land on when Santa Claus arrives.

Then we had the amazing rain of 21 July, when it rained, almost torrentially, from around 1 am until 11 pm. At least one local school was cut off and the kids had to stay overnight because they couldn't get home. At another school, to be precise a primary school on the same road as the secondary school James goes to, firemen had to carry the kids from the school to their waiting parents. On TV there were hilarious pictures of a man trying to slow traffic down because it was splashing water down his drive and into his house. A large part of Worcester (not us) was without electricity for the night, and Lizzie's boyfriend's father, having driven to Bristol, had to turn back on the way home but couldn't get back to Bristol either. I'm not sure where he spent the night. The cricket ground half a mile away from us flooded again; Worcestershire gave up and decided to play the rest of the season outside Worcester. I seem to remember it was around this time last year that Elton John played there, he would have needed a boat this year! The racecourse, a quarter of a mile away, was under water (I think that the technical term is 'heavy going'!). It goes without saying that the road below us, which runs parallel to the river, was flooded and closed, as were the poor sods who live in a row of terraced, and probably uninsurable, houses further along it.

We were safe as we are relatively high up. The day after it rained was even worse. The rain had stopped but, as usual, we got all the extra water the River Severn had collected further upstream, in Shrewsbury and beyond, and Worcestershire became the first county to request assistance from the army. At one stage, both bridges were closed and we were effectively cut off from central Worcester. It was definitely worse than in 2000, and we are very thankful we live on a hill. I blame the Welsh, they should have sent their spare water to Wimbledon earlier in the summer like everywhere else does.

Changing the subject…

Life at work has been a little difficult as my head of department seems to have decided he wants to get rid of me. To be fair, this is nothing personal as he appears to want to drive out everyone and replace them with young, easily-controlled, very junior lecturers. Eight staff have left already and so maybe he's just trying to get into double figures by getting rid of me and one other. It's like living in a Doctor Who story, in which an evil force invades a planet and tries to change all the inhabitants into robots. Come to think of it, he talks a bit like a Dalek. He is Japanese and really only got the job by accident. He was wandering round the department, lost, heavily armed and not entirely convinced the war was over, when he came across the candidates for the headship. They all took one look at him and immediately decided they didn't want the job. He has not been a great success as head of department though. He is totally unable to see any point of view other than his own, is a control freak (or perhaps just a freak), and models his man management technique on the army's policy on deserters in wartime. Furthermore, student numbers are down as he keeps taking gangs of them off to build bridges over the local rivers. But thank God, I'm not a horse. If I were and it was up to him, I'd probably have been in pieces on a ferry to Calais, in a crateful of tins with French labels on a long time ago. On the other hand, being a horse might be quite attractive. Hours and hours hanging around in fields with your mates, eating grass, nuzzling the mares, and sleeping sounds pretty good to me.

Sadly, our dispute degenerated into a full-scale war and, of course, the Japanese have a mixed record on wars. I think that I came out of it best. The upshot was I have some pretty meaningless 'targets', a bit of administration to do, a new laptop and printer/scanner, etc. to help me work (what a hardship!) and I have to invade China. Ok, I made the last one up. But it has turned out quite well, except we now barely talk to each other, which is a bit difficult as we share a course. Although as he doesn't speak English very well, we have never talked much anyway. No matter, I only want to work until we've got Lizzie through university. I must say, though, it never fails to amaze me how seriously people take their work, and how so many people seem to delight in making life difficult in the workplace. I could write a book about all the intrigue and infighting that goes in a university. Actually, I think someone already has.

It is probably true to say that academics are one of the professions most obsessed with their work. I've lost count of the number of conference sessions I've sat through, which have overrun because some sad individual becomes excited by having an audience of double figures. And who assumes we all share his obsessive interest in the development of a harmonised European Union policy on rat-catching, or additives to cat food, or Morris dancing, or something equally obscure. These people are not the worst, they just won't stop talking, but deep down they know no-one is interested, and we are all really here to have a break, see publishers and co-authors, get drunk with old mates from other universities and avoid the weekly shopping trip to Sainsbury's. Oh what a giveaway!

The real bores are the pompous ones who really believe their research on basket weaving in the 17th century is essential for the future of mankind, and say things like, "I'll just have a half please, as I have to do some research when I get home," or, "I was thinking about that in bed last night." I prefer a more practical and audience-friendly approach. The best paper I ever gave was at an American conference in the mid-1990s. I spoke as the sixth and final speaker on a ludicrously overcrowded 90-minute panel, including a talkative Greek who didn't seem to have to breathe like the rest of us. I came on last, just 7 minutes before the end. I simply said, "My paper is entitled 'The Next Mediterranean Enlargement of the European Union - Malta, Cyprus and Turkey?' to which the answer is probably, possibly and not bloody likely," and then sat down. There were three questions, all directed to me, we finished on time and you could almost touch the relief of the audience.

But work is not what it was. We have had so many new staff starting this year it is hard to keep up and easy to get confused. I was caught out when our new head of graduate studies asked me why I was ignoring his email. How was I supposed to know that Angel Sombrera was not a persistent Latin American sex trade worker trying to sell me dirty photographs but was, in fact, him? He'd told me his name was Lou!

The university is in the throes of yet another major reorganisation. 15 years ago, we had half a dozen faculties, but they were too big and so we were broken down to twenty-odd schools. Now schools are too small and we are being reorganised into half a dozen colleges. These are definitely different to faculties because…because…they have a different name presumably. Craziest of all, we are scheduled to move back into our old building, a 12-storey 1960's tower, which we vacated in 2000 because it was deemed 'totally unsuitable' for academic departments. As a former colleague, now departed to the sanity of Warwick University, used to say to me, "There's the real world, and then there's the University of Edgbaston."

But the worst thing is the department is so colourless, mechanical and devoid of character. Even the mad Scotsman in the office opposite mine just mopes around quietly. He occasionally hums 'Flower of Scotland' during departmental meetings, but has given up playing the bagpipes in his office and throwing empty bottles of Glenfiddich through his window at passing Japanese students. Mind you, that is partly because he accidentally threw out a full one last summer and was inconsolable for days. I did try and provoke him by exchanging a copy of 'The Joys of Visiting Japan' for his spare copy of Sitting Bull's biography but it had no effect. In the office next to mine, I now have one of the new automated young female lecturers, who are programmed to act as enthusiastic cheerleaders for anything the head of department suggests. Exam meetings are worse. In the old days they would go on for hours and we'd have to send out for coffee, sandwiches and cigarettes at least twice. We would get at least one good fight, which often came perilously close to physical violence. And someone would insist on arguing a case for giving a 2.1 to someone whose marks were not even close to nearly being good enough, on the grounds that their kitten had trapped its paw in the door as they left for the exam. Or they had suffered temporary memory loss and mistaken their local pub for the examination hall, and had drunk 12 pints of lager before they realised their error, or some such ludicrous story. These days, a list of students' names and degree classification is read out like a roll call at a POW camp, no-one says anything, and the meeting is over in 36 minutes. It is all so dull!

I suppose I'd better say at least something about the family. Anne is still working 18 hours per week in the Eye Unit at the hospital, although she too is thinking about retirement. The hospital seems to be competing with the University of Edgbaston for the public body that makes the most unnecessary and expensive changes in 2007/08. Clare is happily completing her MA in Music (piano) at the Royal Welsh College of Music and Drama in Cardiff. Lizzie is in her first year at UWE in Bristol, following her boyfriend against our advice. She could have gone to Surrey, Swansea or Aberystwyth. James is finishing his GCSEs this year, or possibly starting them. It's hard to tell, he doesn't seem to do much at all to us, but assures us he is going to Sixth Form College next year. I just hope all his classes are in the afternoon. And my eldest daughter, Angie, well she produced another child, Sally, in June. Same father as number two, and is to be seen (mostly) happily pushing a double buggy with a five-month year old and a 19-month year old in it around town. So far, she is coping quite well and her son, aged 5, is doing well at school. He is quite delightful. We took him to the seaside for a week in the summer and managed to pick the only decent week weather-wise of the school holiday. It did make me feel old though, especially when we visited a park I'd first been taken to as a toddler over 50 years ago!

I hope your family is in good health and spirit as we raise a glass (or two) and wish you a merry Christmas and a happy New Year.

DECEMBER 2008

Well, Christmas 2007 was busy and noisy with 12 for lunch, including a five year old, a toddler and a baby, but the year that preceded it was reassuringly dull. On the presents front I excelled myself in the 'joke present for your wife' category by giving Anne a harmonica and a book of instructions on how to play it. Having been healthy over Christmas, I subsequently contracted the family December cold, so I thought, which Anne and Clare had developed into a particularly virulent strain. I responded in my usual way by dosing myself with Lemsip laced with honey and brandy. Sometimes I cut out the Lemsip and honey; what's left does absolutely nothing for the cold but makes me feel drunk enough not to care about it anymore. Consequently, I am afraid I went on to spend New Year's Eve in 'pathetic-male with minor illness mode' and stayed in bed all day watching old videos, coughing, reading, sleeping, and croaking requests for hot drinks. Not rising until 11 pm to see the new year in and cook a ham omelette with little enthusiasm, from mc that is although I don't suppose the ham omelette was terribly enthusiastic about being eaten either! Things got worse, my cold was actually a particularly nasty virus that was going around and I ended up taking two weeks' sick leave.

At least I kept my germs to myself, unlike the martyrs who exist in every workplace and insist on coming in no matter what. Crawling through the snow with two broken legs and a brave smile on their faces, having been run over by a snowplough on the way to work, or heroically trying to stop the flow of blood with paper towels from the staff toilet, having been attacked by a crocodile in the carpark. There are two extreme examples of this type of person where Anne works who will probably have their coffins brought in when they die to be used as coffee tables or desks.

Talking of carparks and therefore cars, I can hardly believe it but it's time for us to start thinking about getting a new one. Having PD allows me to join the Motability scheme, which is a wonderful arrangement whereby I can get a new car every three years with tax, RAC membership, insurance and two dancing girls wearing stockings and suspenders all thrown in for a very modest monthly payment. Oh alright, not the dancing girls then, that was just wishful thinking. The only drawback is that if you break down you have to stand next to one of those horrible orange RAC vans, and pretend it has nothing to do with you for however long it takes to fix your car. To be honest, I'm not really a car person. I think they are at best necessary evils and that future generations will come to regard the early 21st century with amazement as a period in which mankind allowed the motor car a ridiculous amount of dominance. Of course, the driver matters a lot, my dad used to tell the story of a man who was a rotten driver and if ever he got into the driving seat of the family car his kids would all get out and refuse to get back in until their mother was behind the steering wheel.

I suppose it might help if I were a bit more mechanically-minded, but I am afraid you are reading a letter from someone who would answer the question 'what kind of car do you have?' with 'a blue one'. Or if I wanted to be technical 'a light blue one'. The only way I'm ever going to change a wheel is with the help of the Magic Circle. Nor can I comprehend men who love and endlessly clean and polish their cars, what are automatic car-washers for? The only reasons I can see for having a car are:

(a) it gets you from A to B faster than a horse, unless the horse is driving a sports car or, on roller skates in congested areas,

(b) it is a warm and dry place to sit while someone drives you to and from the pub, and,

(c) it means you don't have to travel by bus or train and sit next to someone arranging their social life in great detail on their mobile phone.

And why anyone should want an intimate knowledge of the internal workings of a motor car any more than they would want to be familiar with the insides of a dishwasher or an electric tooth brush is beyond me.

Having said that, I must admit there are occasionally times when I do wish I were more mechanically-minded and, indeed, more practical generally. So many things seem to come in flat boxes these days and have to be put together. I think most shop floor/window displays are totally misleading. For example, those immaculate bedroom displays in MFI ought to be replaced by a dozen cardboard boxes, all open to some degree, with loads of tools scattered on the floor, and a middle-aged man kneeling in the middle of them, with his head in his hands, alternating between sobbing pitifully and swearing loudly at the boxes. And those wonderful-looking combined desks and computer work stations ought to be replaced by a half-full, flat-pack box of desk extension parts and a rickety desk being attacked by a man with an axe, restrained by two men in white coats. That would be a bit more realistic! I look forward to the day when we reach the logical conclusion of purchasing self-assembly furniture, when I go to buy a wardrobe and I am given an axe and directions to the nearest forest.

Indeed, I discovered this year that even things which come fully made can be problematic to buy. We had to replace our washing machine in the summer and wanted a cream one but at the moment a cream washing machine cannot be had anywhere. It is apparently not one of the colours in fashion. I found this mind boggling. How on earth can a washing machine be out of fashion, or in fashion for that matter? It's just there to wash, isn't it? It doesn't cry in its room and complain that no-one will want to dance with it at the school disco if its top is the wrong colour, or sulk for a week because you haven't bought the right designer label trainers for its wheels. Ye gods, whatever next? Fridges with hats on? Punk vacuum cleaners that spit as they vacuum? Somewhat bizarrely, as we spent over £100 between 1 and 3 pm on the particular day we bought a machine, we qualified for a surprise gift in the shape of a full-sized cricket bat, supplied and signed by the players of Worcestershire, a couple of whom were in the shop pretending to be famous. Why they weren't playing cricket somewhere on such a nice day I'm not sure. I wish I had been. Given the stress involved in buying a new washer, and having just about mastered the concept of fashionable washing machines, I thought I did well to keep a straight face whilst accepting the bat. It wasn't easy acting as though receiving a cricket bat as a free gift when you bought a washing machine was the most natural thing in the world. Anne was somewhat less impressed with the gift than me. Although, to be fair to her, she knew which end of the bat to hold and also which way up to hold it, and went on to make 34 not out and take two wickets in an impromptu charity game with the Worcestershire players in the car park. (All proceeds donated to the local Home for Middle- Aged Men Driven Mad by Attempting to Assemble MFI Furniture Society.)

On returning home, I put the cricket bat between the front legs of the horse we were looking after in the hall. Not a real horse, of course, but a rather large rocking horse a friend had asked us to take care of while part of her house is decorated. Nevertheless, although the horse wasn't real, it can still be a little disconcerting, not to say downright alarming, to come downstairs and bump into any sort of horse in the middle of the night. What exactly our friend thought the decorators were going to do with it is not clear. Perhaps she thought they might be tempted to paint a moustache on it, or dress up as clowns and ride the horse bareback as they painted the ceiling?

Work is becoming a bit of a struggle but I am determined to carry on for as long as I can. At least I have had the satisfaction of seeing off our Japanese head of department, who has now passed the poisoned chalice on to a much nicer Englishman. And, as all outgoing heads of department are wont to do, he has departed for foreign climes to hide from all the enemies, a record number in his case, he made while he was head of department.

Going back to my illness, the trouble is that as soon as I resolve one medical problem, another seems to crop up. My latest affliction is that I've started to stutter. This is not good for a lecturer as it obviously makes it difficult for students, particularly overseas MA students, to understand me. Although, come to think of it, they didn't understand me when I didn't stutter because most of them don't speak English. These days, our only requirement as far as English language skills are concerned is the ability to write 'I promise to pay the University of Edgbaston 8,000 pounds'. And this is still more stringent than some other universities where prospective students only have to be able to write '10,000 pounds', they charge more than we do, and are prepared to provide an interpreter to write the rest, for a suitable additional fee.

The most amazing thing that's happened at work this year is Mad Rab, the Scotsman in the office opposite me, has got married and not only is he very happy, he is a changed man. He now manages to stay sober until well into the afternoon, has stopped calling the head of department 'Jimmy', and incredibly, he now puts his empty cans of Iron Bru into a recycling bin instead of filling them with sand and throwing them at passing undergraduates. He also keeps going on about bairns, or possibly burns. It's not clear to me whether he's thinking of starting a family, has discovered an interest in Scottish poetry, or is developing a tendency towards pyromania. In any case, it's as well to keep the matches away from him, as if he as much as breathes on a naked light after 3 o'clock in the afternoon half the campus is likely to go up in flames.

I just hope the marriage lasts. If it doesn't he'll be heartbroken and get depressed. The last time he got depressed, he locked himself in the physics department's seminar room and wouldn't come out until he'd consumed the two crates of Glenfiddich he'd taken in with him. It took nearly two days. It wouldn't have been so bad but the entire physics department were in there having a meeting at the time, and by the time they got out they were severely traumatised. Living with the threat of being hit by a flying whisky bottle was bad enough, but what really sent them over the edge was Rab's non-stop playing of, and singing along to, Jimmy Logan's 'Hogmanay Hits and Other Scottish Dirges' on his portable music system. In the end they had to amalgamate the departments of physics and psychiatry, in the hope the two halves of the new department would help each other. It seems to have worked well. Last year they ran a very successful international conference 'Physicists And Their Mothers: The Oedipus Complex Revisited' and preparations are already well underway for a second. 'Freud, Black Holes And The Big Bang: Is Academic Research Just An Opportunity To Dress Up In Dirty Old White Lab Coats And Ask Women To Lie Down On Couches?'

Turning to the family. It's not been a terribly good year for Anne. Both her parents, now approaching their mid-80s, have had spells in hospital this year and are not well. Angie continues to surprise us. She is very well organised and seems quite content to stay at home looking after her three kids, now aged 6, 2 and 1, whom she is bringing up very well. Clare completed her MA at the Royal Welsh College of Drama and Music and has taken a job, for at least a year, as a teaching assistant at Wells Cathedral School. Wells is a lovely place, we spent a weekend there, if a little inaccessible. Lizzie is doing OK. She is in her second year at UWE in Bristol, but has split with her boyfriend of three years whom she went to Bristol (against our wishes) to be with. James managed to get a reasonable collection of GCSEs and seems to be doing well at Sixth Form College, mainly because he is now only doing subjects he likes. I continue, slightly worse, and I think early retirement on health grounds is not far away.

And, finally, heard on the radio during the international banking crisis earlier in the year:

"And bad news from Japan, the origami bank has just folded."

So, it's goodnight and merry Christmas from him,

And goodnight and merry Christmas from her.

NOVEMBER 2009

Some serious stuff and big changes in 2009, and so this year's letter is correspondingly more reflective, and boring, in places. The tone was set by Christmas 2008, which was a somewhat muted affair as Anne's mother entered her sixth week in hospital, and so there was an empty seat at the table. She did go home for a week or so in January, but she deteriorated again and so was readmitted to hospital, where she died on 1 March.

More big adjustment is to follow in 2010 as I finally decided enough was enough and I will retire on ill-health grounds in the autumn. I ought to be pretty pleased with myself really. When I was diagnosed in December 1995, the consultant told me I could expect to work for five to ten more years and I've managed 14, admittedly as something of a passenger for the last two to three. So I've kept going well past my sell-by date. The nature of my job has helped, of course. I would have been well and truly up the creek without a paddle had I been a bricklayer or an acrobat or, indeed, a man who travelled to work in a rowing boat and had lost his oars.

I shall be glad to be out of it actually. The department has changed out of all recognition. Although in one respect, the physical working environment, it is vastly improved. We've moved back into the tower block and surprise, surprise, they've thrown lots of money at it and most of the offices are wonderful. There is none of the politically correct equality that we had in our last building (rabbit hutch-sized offices for all). My office is in one of the professorial wings and is huge, two desks, a table and four chairs, and still room for a snooker table, an armchair and cat-swinging competitions. And the corridors are so wide and bright, there are photocopiers and kitchen areas with fridges, microwaves, etc. in both wings on every floor, plentiful lifts that work, and even a Starbucks coffee shop on the ground floor. Working there is also made easier by the fact that the department is located on the 2nd and 3rd floors and the teaching rooms are on the 1st floor.

Of course, it means I am no longer opposite the mad Scotsman and so it is very quiet. He is in a cupboard a few doors away, complaining bitterly all the time about the small size of his office. Now he's no longer semi-conscious by 2 pm every day, he tends to notice where he is and react accordingly. He leaves his door open so everyone can see how small his office is, although it's not working at the moment because the secretaries have got fed up of looking at him and have blocked his door with a Christmas tree. I'm not sure why exactly he wants a bigger office, it's not as if he can practise tossing the caber in there like he did in his old office. He's not allowed to do that anywhere on campus since the incident with the caber, the undergraduate nun, the Vice-Chancellor's cat and a tub of I-Can't-Believe-It's-Not-Butter last January. Don't ask, suffice it to say he was lucky to get away with a suspended sentence, is now blacklisted by the Vatican, the RSPCA and the

Margarine Producers Association, and the cat is still in therapy nearly 12 months later.

However, the department is not so much quiet nowadays, more like a ghost town. All the professors are in management meetings and all the junior staff are out protesting about the impending closure of the sociology department. I don't know what all the fuss is about. It has closed twice already during my time at Edgbaston, the first time it more-or-less closed itself when all the staff left. But sociologists are like an infestation; you keep thinking you've gotten rid of them and then they reappear. They are never going to be a protected species like physicists or university administrators, but are never going to be completely wiped out either because they have developed their own methods of surviving.

Fortunately, it wasn't just endings in 2009. There were some beginnings. In July we went to a wedding, and it was a good one. The setting was glorious, a country hotel with weather to match, although I am not quite sure how I ended up being sat at a table with an air hostess, three policemen and a retired professional rugby player (Wakefield Trinity). We stayed in a hotel 15 miles away in Clitheroe, near Blackburn, which is one of those places you've sort of heard of but never really thought existed. It is most accurately described as a typical, small and quiet Lancashire/Yorkshire market town with lots of pubs. For some reason it also has a castle, I'm not sure why, it is difficult enough to find Clitheroe, let alone attack it, and any attacker would have to go through most of the town centre to get to the castle. Perhaps this is the castle's best defence because the town itself is full of charity shops and hairdressers, which together probably accounted for up to a quarter of the shops. I imagine any attacking force would be overwhelmed by the many bargains and opportunities for a decent haircut and a drink in one of the pubs. "Put down the battering ram, lads, and sod the castle and the raping and pillaging, let's go and have a perm and a pint, and see if we can find a few bargains."

The wedding was in a hotel rather than a church, which seems to be the way these days. In my youth, a large part of my social life revolved around our local C. of E. church. Firstly, from the age of eight to 17 I was a member of the choir. This was quite a commitment but we had a laugh and used to play lots of pranks. The organist, Mrs Watson, who was probably born as an old lady and was surely never a child, used to disapprove strongly and glare at us through a mirror she had on the organ (she played with her back to us). That was when she could because at every opportunity we would twist the mirror so it wasn't directed at us. I eventually graduated into being a server (altar boy) which was quite a responsible job. In fact, I was always the senior server unless John Samuels was serving. Only God and the vicar outranked the Samuels in our church.

In addition, I became a member of the Church Lads Brigade, which was organised very much on military lines. By this, I don't mean that we hung about outside Catholic churches causing trouble, or fought holy wars against the Patels who ran the local Indian takeaway but rather that we had uniforms and ranks, and lost no opportunity to go on parade and march about a bit, especially on Remembrance Sunday. I eventually became a sergeant. The church also ran a youth club, which was very fashionable at the time. We went on a daytrip once. The vicar was also chaplain of the local borstal and so some borstal boys came. One of them told us 11 different ways to break into and steal a car. Sensibly, I have never acted on this information.

But I wasn't especially religious and not everything I did was with the church. In particular, it was wonderful being a kid in a village surrounded on three sides by countryside and every summer was an adventure. There were few restrictions placed on us in those days as we rampaged around the fields and country lanes to the west of the village. I can still remember the sense of freedom and adventure. I feel sorry for kids today, huddled over their computer screens, overprotected and overfed by parents who see paedophiles, drunken drivers and drug dealers around every corner. They may be able to travel the world through cyberspace whilst we lived in a much smaller world, but at least our world was real and we were free. After a few years the lanes became too familiar and we ventured further afield. One summer, while exploring beyond the lanes, we discovered a stretch of water, all that was left of the 'old' River Don as the river was re-routed in the 17th century to reduce flooding. The great attraction of this lake/river was that it was the best place we knew for collecting bulrushes. God knows why we small boys valued bulrushes so much, but they were highly prized, and we would go to great lengths to obtain them and then hide them. They grew in abundance on the mud island that had appeared in the centre of the old Don. It was true that you had to cross some barbed wire and wade out in up to four feet of water to get to this island, but that was merely a minor inconvenience. You were supposed to soak the bulrushes in petrol and then set them alight. To this day, I have no idea what possible purpose this highly dangerous activity was for but, of course, we had no access to petrol and being caught playing with matches was a serious offence in the eyes of our parents. And so, we hid and hoarded the bulrushes, and forgot about them.

Another year we explored the other end of the village beyond the recreation ground. This was the site of the (by then closed) pit and, more importantly, two sets of slagheaps, the 'black hills', where we played. These were very extensive. The ones to the front of the pit were fairly small and low-lying, with the exception of one very big one, and this provided us with our very own all year round skiing, or rather sledging, facility. We kids came down the slope on sledges, pieces of tin and squashed cardboard boxes. There was even one lunatic who used to come down on a bike. This was absolute madness and it's a wonder he didn't seriously injure himself. My friends and I certainly never tried it. The 'black hills' to the back of the pit were much higher and more extensive, like a mini-mountain range and we had great fun climbing and exploring them. Although the Aberfan disaster must have happened around this time, and I'm sure that there were notices warning us off, we never thought of this activity as being dangerous, although it probably was.

The Aberfan disaster was the collapse of a spoil tip ('black hill') onto the Welsh village of Aberfan in 1966. The local junior school was buried. A total of five teachers and 109 school children died, and a further 30 were killed elsewhere in the village, resulting in a total death toll of 144.

But accidents also happened underground and, when I was 6 or 7, my dad had a serious accident at the pit where he worked. The village pit had closed in 1956 because of flooding, and all the men were transferred to other pits with special buses were laid on to take them there. The arrival and departure of the 'pit buses' around an hour before the time of a shift change were a regular feature of our lives. The thing I actually remember most about my dad's time as a miner, was him bringing my sister and I something nice home, usually a Mars Bar each, hidden in his snap tin, when he came home in the morning. He worked 'nights regular' because it was better paid, I presume. A snap tin was an oblong tin all the men had, in which they carried their 'snap' (food), often bread and jam or bread and dripping. For some reason the cans had to be airtight and, of course, they also took flasks of tea to drink, but obviously not cigarettes, which were strictly banned for fear of explosion.

My dad worked on the coalface of the Yorkshire Main at Edlington about 10 miles away. On that fateful night he was lucky not to lose either one leg, both legs or his life. He later told me the following. He operated an electric coal-cutting machine and had a new man with him. My dad got in front of the machine to clear away some debris and somehow the machine was accidentally switched on and scythed his legs from under him. I don't remember much about it, but my mother had the shock of her life when there was a knock on the door at 4 am from my dad's friends, who had brought his clothes and other possessions. This was usually a sign that a woman's husband was dead, which I think they thought my dad was as good as.

He was in hospital for a very long time, first a specialist hospital in Sheffield, then a spell recuperating in Doncaster hospital, and finally weeks at home on crutches. I think he also spent a fortnight by the sea at a miners' rest home or something similar. The whole process took over a year. I remember my dad returning home on crutches and how happy we were as he hopped from the ambulance to the house.

Virtually the whole street came out to welcome him. When my dad recovered, he opted not to return to the coalface, indeed, he would never work underground again, and instead he was given a surface job by the NCB. But he could not settle and soon left the mines behind him. For a while, he worked as an overhead crane driver at International Harvesters at Doncaster, and then as a fitter's mate in one of the two boatyards that flourished alongside the canal at nearby Thorne. He eventually moved on to factory work and spent the last years of his working life employed at Youngs Seafood, also in Thorne. I used to call Youngs the family firm as, at various times, they employed not only my father but also my mother, my sister, a cousin, an aunt, two uncles and, indeed, myself during a summer vacation from university one year.

So, to the family news. Angie continues in much the same vein. Her son (7) is doing well at school and the two little girls (3 & 2) are developing into a comedy double-act. Clare is continuing her tour of Celtic music colleges and began a course in piano accompaniment, which is what she now wants to do, at the Royal Scottish Academy of Music and Drama in Glasgow in September. Lizzie is in her final year of university at UWE in Bristol and is 21 soon, how time flies, and is living in a flat in a spot many would kill for, at the top of Park Street for those of you who know Bristol. James continues at Worcester Sixth Form College where he is currently completely wrapped up in rehearsals for the College's annual musical in December. It's 'Sweeney Todd' this year, in which he's playing the title role. It's nice to have one of our offspring on the stage for a change, Clare and Lizzie both played the piano in the band for the annual musical when they were at the College. Finally, Anne, like me, has experienced big changes at work and is finding many of the staff she has worked with for some years have retired, or are going to do so quite soon, and is increasingly inclined to join them.

Well, that's about it for this year, sorry this is such a dull letter. To compensate, I attach an innovation to my Christmas letters, a quiz for Christmas! I shall send you the answers next year, but if you can't wait, email me and I'll send them by email.

Merry Quiz-mas and a Happy New Year!

XMAS QUIZ - QUESTIONS

Twenty Questions and 1 point per question

Round - 1 - TRADITIONS

1. Which member of the Royal Family (past or present) is particularly associated with many aspects of Christmas as we celebrate it today?
2. The Christmas tree in Trafalgar Square is traditionally provided by the capital city of which country
3. Which two vegetables (excluding carrots) are normally served as part of a Christmas dinner?
4. In which decade in the 19th century were the first Christmas cards sent?
5. How did good King Wenceslas like his pizza?

Round – 2 - BOOKS AND TELEVISION

6. What gift does Father Christmas give to the boy near the end of the film, `The Snowman?'

7. Complete the first line of the poem 'The Night Before Christmas'. It was the night before Christmas, and all through the house…

8. Who appeared as Doctor Who for the very first time in the 2005 Christmas Special 'The Christmas Invasion?"

9. What is the name of Scrooge's former business partner?

10. Who narrates the 1892 short story that centres on a blue carbuncle being found in the neck of a Christmas goose?

Round – 3 - MUSIC

11. Who composed the music for the ballet 'The Nutcracker'?

12. Which has been the only group to have had four Christmas number ones?

13. What colour was Elvis Presley's Christmas in 1964?

14. What was Slade's Noddy Holder's granny up and doing with the rest, despite telling him that the old songs are the best?

15. According to Jimmy Boyd's 1952 hit, what did he see his mummy doing with Santa under the Christmas tree?

Round - 4 - POT POURRI

16. Which carol am I describing?

Omnipotent supreme being who gives respite to jolly well-mannered males.

17. In which ocean is Christmas Island located?

18. What would you call Father Christmas if you saw him at the South Pole?

19. Which one of the following was NOT at number one in the charts for Cliff Richard on Christmas Day:

Mistletoe and Wine or Savour's Day or Millennium Prayer?

And finally, an anagram:

20. 'Smart heretics' and 'Merriest chats' are both anagrams of which two words?

DECEMBER 2010

Sorry but there is no Christmas letter this year. I have not been very well. To compensate for this tragic loss of Christmas reading material/toilet paper, I am sending the answers to last year's quiz for your entertainment.

Merry Christmas

XMAS QUIZ – ANSWERS (WITH QUESTIONS)

Twenty Questions and 1 point per question

Round - 1 - TRADITIONS

1. Which member of the Royal Family (past or present) is particularly associated with many aspects of Christmas as we celebrate it today?
    PRINCE ALBERT

2. The Christmas tree in Trafalgar Square is traditionally provided by the capital city of which country?
    NORWAY (CAPITAL CITY IS OSLO)

The Trafalgar Square Christmas tree has been an annual gift since 1947 to the people of Britain by the city of Oslo as a token of gratitude for British support to Norway during the Second World War.

3. Which two vegetables (excluding carrots) are normally served as part of a Christmas dinner?

SPROUTS AND PARSNIPS

4. In which decade in the 19th century were the first Christmas cards sent?

THE 1840s (I'll take the 1830s or 1850s as well)

The first Christmas cards were sent in 1843 by Sir Henry Cole, a senior civil servant.

5. How did good King Wenceslas like his pizza?

Deep PAN, crisp (and even).

Good King Wenceslas last looked out
On the Feast of Stephen
When the snow lay round about
DEEP PAN, CRISP AND EVEN

OR (AN ALTERNATIVE VERSION)

Good King Wencelas last ate out
On the Feast of Stephen

Bought a pizza to take out
DEEP PAN, CRISP (AND EVEN)

Round – 2 - BOOKS AND TELEVISION

6. What gift does Father Christmas give to the boy near the end of the film, "The Snowman?

A SCARF

7. Complete the first line of the poem 'The Night Before Christmas'. It was the night before Christmas, and all through the house…

Not a creature was stirring, not even a mouse

8. Who appeared as Doctor Who for the very first time in the 2005 Christmas Special 'The Christmas Invasion?"
DAVID TENNANT.

9. What is the name of Scrooge's former business partner?
JACOB MARLEY

10. Who narrates the 1892 short story that centres on a blue carbuncle being found in the neck of a Christmas goose?
DOCTOR WATSON - It's a Sherlock Holmes short story.

Round – 3 - MUSIC

11. Who composed the music for the ballet 'The Nutcracker'?
Tchaikovsky

12. Which has been the only group to have had four Christmas number ones?
The Beatles. The songs were 'I Wanna Hold Your Hand' (1963), 'I Feel Fine' (1964), 'Day Tripper'/'We Can Work It Out' (1965) and 'Hello-Goodbye' (1967).

13. What colour was Elvis Presley's Christmas in 1964?
BLUE
Elvis had a hit with 'Blue Christmas' that year.

14. What was Slade's Noddy Holder's granny up and doing with the rest, despite telling him that the old songs are the best?
ROCK'N'ROLLING

15. According to Jimmy Boyd's 1952 hit, what did he see his mummy doing with Santa under the Christmas tree?
KISSING
The song was 'I Saw Mummy Kissing Santa Claus'.

Round - 4 - POT POURRI

16. Which carol am I describing?

Omnipotent supreme being who gives respite to jolly well-mannered males.

'God Rest Ye Merry Gentlemen'

17. In which ocean is Christmas Island located?
INDIAN OCEAN

18. What would you call Father Christmas if you saw him at the South Pole?
LOST (OR SOMETHING SIMILAR) – HE LIVES AT THE NORTH POLE.

19. Which one of the following was NOT at number one in the charts for Cliff Richard on Christmas Day?
Mistletoe and Wine or Saviour's Day or Millennium Prayer
MILLENNIUM PRAYER .
It was number 1 the week before Christmas but was knocked off the top spot in Christmas week by Westlife.

And finally, an anagram:

20. 'Smart heretics' and 'Merriest chats' are both anagrams of which two words?
CHRISTMAS TREE

DECEMBER 2011

Sorry there was no Christmas letter in 2010, you may have not even got a card. Although Christmas and Christmas Day themselves were fine, I really was not very well. My PD symptoms got much worse and I began to go downhill fairly rapidly, becoming virtually housebound, chair-bound almost. I had still been doing a little teaching at the end of 2009, but in 2010 I didn't go into work at all and eventually took early retirement on ill health grounds at the end of September. Things did not improve at the beginning of this year and so I decided to have brain surgery, which took place in January. I had an operation called deep brain stimulation which is quite long (9am-5 pm) and involves electrodes being attached to the brain, with an electric current passed through, powered by a battery implanted underneath the skin on the chest, a bit like a heart pace- maker; the battery has to be replaced every seven to eight years.

There then follows several difficult months as the brain adjusts to the implant and you experiment with your drug regime. The idea is you end up taking fewer drugs. It was a rough ride and we did not really get it right until August, but I am now much improved and have a life again. The brain stimulation gives me a basic level of mobility even when I have taken no drugs, for example, during the night. I can do things around the house again, such as cooking and basic housework, I go shopping alone on the bus, and have even travelled independently by train to Edgbaston. Anne and I have had a couple of three-night breaks in hotels and hope to book a proper holiday in 2012. About the only things I don't do is drive and play the piano, although, I couldn't play the piano before I had Parkinson's and it is possible I will give driving a go eventually. Of course, I still do have bad days and I still do not sleep very well but, on balance, I am much better than I was.

I had another spell in hospital later, after the operation to try and sort out my drug regime. The Queen Elizabeth Hospital at Edgbaston has become my favourite holiday destination. This year's hospital stays were relatively uneventful, apart from the statutory old man repeatedly telling his life story. He was, I increasingly believe, one of several actually employed by the hospital as a sleeping aid to other patients. I also played a game of cricket using a rolled-up magazine and tennis ball with two other patients. Unfortunately, after several stoppages 'nurse stopped play' and a pitch invasion by the lady with the tea trolley, the game had to be abandoned as a draw as the fourth patient, acting as umpire from his bed, was still unconscious after his operation and couldn't give anyone out. At least, this was better than in cricket in the Intensive Care Unit where 'retired, dead' is the most common way of getting out, and in the amputees' unit where it is virtually impossible to get an lbw (leg before wicket) decision.

A sign of my recovery is that I have started to take an interest in the European Union again. In particular, I have been much exercised by the Euro zone crisis. Why exactly we should expect Italy, the country that agrees to everything European but implements nothing, and gave us spaghetti, which is impossible to eat without looking disgusting, to break the habit of a lifetime and act responsibly is beyond me. And the Greeks are even worse. Greece has been going downhill since the demise of Aristotle. The only way to a long-term solution is to dynamite Italy and Greece *pour encourager les autres* (to encourage the others), kick out Spain and Portugal until they stop kipping in the afternoon, kick out the Irish until they know their place and stop winning the Eurovision Song Contest, and start the Euro zone all over again with Germany and a few sensible countries in it.

I have also been sorting out some old photos, which has made me think of my childhood. In my early years, my weekends were devoted to visiting my two family groups, one led by and based on the home of each grandmother, and each group had a rich cast of characters. Saturday was our day at my paternal grandma's. Her house smelled, in a nice way, of food. She cooked in an old-fashioned oven powered by the fire next to it. My granddad was a retired miner so she got her coal for next to nothing, and her dinners tasted like nothing I've ever eaten since. Real food cooked by the heat from a real fire and with a real taste. She was a small woman with an infectious laugh, and came out with the occasional great line, like when she told us my dad's cough would be much reduced "if only he'd start smoking tipped cigarettes." On another occasion, when her nephew, and lodger, who was deaf and dumb, wanted to marry a deaf and dumb woman, she opposed the marriage on the grounds that she was "buggered if she was going to have two of them living in her house."

Apart from looking after her family, she had one other passion. Betting on the horses. And horseracing was something she knew a lot about. I remember every Saturday everything stopped at 5 pm while she listened to the racing results, to see if she'd won. Even when I visited her when she was in her eighties, it was not unusual to find the house empty, the door unlocked (she never locked her door) and a note saying 'Gone to bookies. Back soon'. As far as I can remember, the only time I've ever been in a bookmaker's has been to collect her.

My paternal grandfather didn't make his appearance until after the pubs shut. He was a retired miner and only said one thing to me: "Never work down t'pit, lad." He died when I was 16, when his liver finally lost its battle with the incoming alcohol. I very much regret that I was never old enough to go to the pub with him. Nor obviously did I see him in his younger days when he used to play the piano in the pub for beer money, and was prone to disappearing for a few days. No-one ever found out where he went. And to this day, I don't know for sure if his first name was Michael or Martin.

My maternal grandmother's family was perhaps slightly less entertaining but more plentiful. I lacked a maternal grandfather, as he had died in the 1940s. He was a rather severe looking man; I have one photo of him. He was disappointed at fathering only daughters and kept and raced greyhounds. Not personally, of course, but against other greyhounds. He was from a Dutch family of around a dozen, half born in Holland and the other half (including him) in England. I was never quite sure what happened to all my

Dutch relatives. I think they may have got bored and gone back to Holland. Certainly, I never knew them.

My grandma had 12 younger brothers and sisters, and I was always getting introduced to relatives I had never met before. We used to arrive about 12 noon and I spent most of the time until lunch playing in the house, avoiding the rather vicious cat that lived under the table. It was prone to scratch any living creature that came within five feet of it, except when it was busy giving birth to the litter after litter of kittens it produced in the shed. In the feline world the cat was a whore. After lunch we sat on the tiny front lawn, it was always summer, and I played in a paddling pool while my mother's younger sisters played their records. I still blame them for my embarrassing partiality to Cliff Richard. At some point a man on a bicycle with refrigerated containers on either side blew a whistle and we all trooped over to buy cupfuls of ice-cream. This was high living for a three- or four-year-old, Cliff, ice-cream and a paddling pool. It didn't get any better than that, and, in truth, probably never has.

However, my earliest detailed recollection is the shops near where I lived when I was at infants' school. Indeed, the son of the local grocer around the corner soon became my best friend but our friendship didn't last. I was temporarily banned from his house after I killed their budgie. This was totally accidental but they were very angry about it. Joey, as the budgie was called, had an endearing habit of perching on my friend's model train as it whizzed around his model railway track. I tried to step over it but stepped on it instead, with a fatal result: a broken train and a squashed budgie. The story probably ran for days in the 'Grocers' Daily': Budgie in Fatal Train Accident, Police Question Boy in Budgie-Stamping Incident,

RSPCA Condemn Budgie Atrocity, etc. It was only a bloody budgie, you'd think I'd murdered my friend's sister! However, things were never the same for either me, or obviously the budgie, after the tragedy and I drifted apart from my friend soon afterwards.

The other main shop of interest to me was the corner sweetshop. This was run by Mrs. Brown, who seemed to hate children. Certainly, she would never serve us if there were adults waiting, and she was quick to throw us out if we were noisy or took too long choosing our sweets. God knows how she ended up running a sweetshop. I can only assume she had mass-murderer pretensions and intended to poison the sweets one day.

There was also a newsagent who supplied us with our comics, 'Bunty' and eventually 'Jackie' for my sister, 'The Victor' and 'The Rover' for me and, of course, for all of us 'The Beano', 'Dandy', 'Topper' and 'Beezer'. The boys' comics were full of war stories in which the Germans were always called Fritz and the Japanese always shouted "Banzai!". My God, talk about racial/racist stereotypes! There was one particularly ludicrous story set in the Indian subcontinent where the hero had a side-kick who was a seven foot native, who used to set about the Japanese with a cricket bat shouting 'Clickey ba!' Personally I would have preferred a gun, but this giant was apparently impervious to bullets and so didn't need one. He probably went on to open for Sri Lanka at Lords. 'Well, Brian, this chap certainly has an unorthodox stance, and seems to hit the slip fielders more than the ball…"

And there were the sporting heroes. The great Wilson who was hundreds of years old, it was never clear what his exact age was, who used to run in old fashioned kit and disappear mysteriously at the end. One of my favourites was Alf Tupper, the "Tough of the Track", who would eat a fish and chip supper, work all night repairing his motorbike (whoever sold him that saw him coming, it was always breaking down), ride it 200 miles in pouring rain, pausing only to stop a runaway train, capture an escaped crocodile and lead the British curling team to a gold medal in the Winter Olympics. Oh alright, I made the last three things up. He'd eat more fish and chips, before beating the snobs and winning the race, despite them nailing his running shoes to the starting line while his feet were still in them, and setting dogs on him on the back straight. There was also a goalkeeper who never conceded a goal, every week it looked as though he had but it would turn out that the referee had blown his whistle for the end of the game just before the ball crossed the line, or the ball had gone in through a hole in the side netting, or the match had been abandoned because the Martians had invaded, or something equally ludicrous. Finally, there was a story that particularly captured my dad's imagination. It was set in a future where football had been made illegal and it was about a secret attempt to revive the game.

I also occasionally read my sister's comics, especially the Four Marys who I was pleased to see recently are still at St. Elmo's, even though they are now in their 50s or 60s. Their teachers are still going strong despite being well over a hundred years old. Perhaps their headmistress ought to get together with the great Wilson. But the leading comics were 'The Beano' and 'The Dandy'. The latter I remember less well, except for Desperate Dan and his cow pies and Corky the Cat. 'The Beano' was full of the most amazing characters, Dennis the Menace, Minnie the Minx, Rodger the Dodger, the Bash

Street Kids: Danny, Fattie, Smiffy, Plug. All of whom I vividly recollect. 'The Topper' and 'Beezer' were less memorable, except for the Numskulls and Tom, Dick and Harry with their amazing hair, which stood up on their heads apparently unsupported. I knew a barmaid in Cardiff years later with hair just like that.

Changing the subject, it was a curiously television-free Christmas last year. The only TV I remember watching was a bizarre late-night film in the early hours. I was just flicking through the channels before going to bed when I came across what I thought was an old episode of 'Kojak'. It turned out to be a weird film full of famous people. Dean Martin, Sammy Davis Junior (who the hell was Sammy Davis Senior?) and Burt Reynolds were in it, plus many quite familiar faces I can't name. I couldn't work it out and became even more confused when Shirley MacLean and another famous American actress turned up dressed as nuns and began punching people. Jaws from the Bond movies appeared and hurled Telly Savalas over a roof. We were apparently in the middle of a general fight scene - I'm not making this up, by the way. By then, Jackie Chan of 'Shanghai Nights' fame was kung-fu fighting with all-comers, eventually helped by Burt Reynolds. When Frank Sinatra pulled up in a car I gave up and went to bed. It is truly amazing what they put on in the early hours. I think the oddest thing I've come across is an entire channel devoted to the old western series 'Bonanza' (go on, admit it, the theme music is going through your head, isn't it?). The trouble was they only seemed to have about ten episodes and so it got a bit repetitive.

But I digress. What news from the Redmond clan in 2011? Well, Anne continues to work part-time as a nurse in the eye department at Worcester hospital, but finds the greater use of technology and decreased contact with patients increasingly at odds with her view of what nursing should be about. She is looking forward to retirement, probably in 2013, although she will miss her long drives around the hospital carparks, looking for a space. Angie continues to live quite close, with her partner and three children, although in a different house. She has moved to a bigger place as her original house was very small. Clare completed her second Master's degree, this time in piano accompaniment at the Royal Scottish Academy of Music and Drama in Glasgow, in 2011. We went up for the graduation ceremony, which was really rather nice, with a piper and an opera singer amongst other things. She is still living in Glasgow, working as a pianist with various choirs, singers and other musicians, and also teaching and playing concerts. It's a bit precarious but she loves it. Lizzie is now back living at home. She has got a part-time job at Lloyds Bank and started a two-year part time Master's degree at the University of Edgbaston in September. It's pretty hard going for her but hopefully will pay dividends in the end. And as one returns home, another departs. James is now an undergraduate at the University of Sussex in Brighton, where he started in September, having got good 'A' Level results after his somewhat mixed school career.

But I shall end this year, like a repeat of 'Have I Got News for You', with two stories I came across a few months ago, which are both presumably true.

First, I read this in a newspaper on the way into work on the train in May:

'A married teacher embarked on a year-long affair with a... pupil...jurors heard. The pair...allegedly met once a week for 'music practice' during which the girl, a talented percussionist, performed sex acts on him. She was told to keep playing the xylophone during the incidents so that anyone passing did not disturb them.'

I'll never be able to listen to Patrick Moore playing the xylophone on the radio again!

Second, there was a story on the internet (also in May) about a Spanish tetraplegic, who was stopped on a motorway near Madrid by police, as he travelled 'at considerable speed' in a wheelchair he controlled with his chin. He had apparently got lost while looking for a brothel. What's puzzling me is not so much how he got on the motorway but what exactly was he planning to do when he got to the brothel?

I like to end with a mystery.

Have a good Christmas and, unlike the man in the wheelchair, I hope you find what you are looking for, and don't get arrested!

Keep smiling.

Nil desperandum.

NOVEMBER 2012

Christmas approaches once again. I can only hope it is more relaxing than last year, which degenerated into an exercise in mass catering. We had 11 to feed on Christmas Day, 14 on Boxing Day and 12 on New Year's Day. Consequently, we seemed to spend much of our time in the supermarket and the kitchen. Actually, this year might be just as hectic, albeit for a different reason. Angie is expecting her fourth child on 29th December. We don't have any potential names yet, but I do hope that Angie doesn't take her inspiration from the recent US presidential election. What sort of mother looks at her baby and thinks "I'm going to call him Mitt" and Barack Obama sounds like an instruction to heckle his speeches. And did you know that Mitt's eldest son is called Tagg? Does he have granddaughters called Mitta and Taggina, I wonder? The mind boggles! Do American parents dislike their children or do they all follow Johnny Cash's 'A Boy Named Sue' philosophy?

But at least I have so far avoided antagonising more blind people during the run up to Christmas this year. Whilst I was Christmas shopping in 2011, I stopped suddenly in the street to get something out of my pocket and a blind man and his dog walked into the back of me. We all nearly ended up in a heap on the floor. Then on the way home on the bus, a blind woman sat next to me and I nearly poked her dog's eyes out with my walking stick. Almost a case of the blind leading the blind. The problem is the really good thing about using a walking stick is it encourages people to give you a wide berth, which is probably just as well in my case but unfortunately this does not appear to apply to blind people. They presumably tend to make the conflicting assumption that everyone will get out of their way, especially the 'look at me, I can go as fast as you if I wave my stick in front of me' types. Come to think of it, the man who tunes our piano is blind and, apart from some initial difficulty in finding the piano and several false starts on the settee, he seems to manage perfectly well. Also, on the bright side, I've had no problem with deaf people or wheelchair users so far. But the pavements can be as dangerous as the roads, and someone told me there are many more psychopaths around than there used to be and I should be wary of them. Come to think of it, he may have said cycle paths...

The only safe way to travel may seem to be by wheelchair, although this can cause problems if you get out of your wheelchair. We discovered this on holiday in Ireland when we observed a man getting out of a wheelchair to go into a shop. Two young nuns were walking by and became very excited. They immediately declared that the man walking was a miracle. Within 24 hours, the site of the 'miracle' (a bemused butcher's shop) had been upgraded to a holy shrine and within 72 hours, the first pilgrims arrived. Within a week there were calls for the butcher to be made a saint. At this point the butcher, driven by complaints from his regular customers that the pilgrims had bought up all the pork pies in the hope of finding one with the face of the Virgin Mary drawn on it, came forward with the man who owned the wheelchair. He still couldn't walk properly and the shrine was downgraded to a 'site where there was nearly a miracle' which reduced the flow of pilgrims considerably.

However, apart from collisions with blind people, in general, my health has been quite good this year. My operation in January 2011 led to improvements, which have continued throughout 2012. The operation seems to have given me a basic level of mobility and has allowed me to reduce my drug intake. I still have difficult times of the day, particularly first thing in the morning and late afternoon, but these are manageable and I have developed ways of dealing with them. We even managed to have a holiday in 2012, two weeks on the Scillies in early September. I had to pace myself but I did a lot of walking and getting on and off of boats, in order to visit the smaller islands, of course. I didn't just do it for the hell of it. The weather was surprisingly good, it barely rained at all, although it turned a bit cold the last few days.

It's funny how distances to holiday destinations shrink as you get older. There was a time when going to Cleethorpes, the nearest seaside 'resort' to the village I grew up in, was a major journey. Whereas now it is barely 45 minutes away from my home village on the motorway. It was to feature fairly regularly in the first 18 years of my life and hardly at all for the rest of it. For many years my dad's working men's club ran an annual daytrip, usually to Cleethorpes, although occasionally we went to Blackpool. There were 20 or so buses and parts of the village became a ghost town for the day. Nowadays, of course, they would be busloads of burglars waiting at Cleethorpes to descend on the village but not back then. There were probably some people who didn't even bother to lock their doors, not that they had anything worth stealing. There were separate buses for children and adults, and the build-up began the night before with the making of the sandwiches. By the time we eventually got on the buses we kids were highly excited and highly excitable. Looking back, our parents knew exactly what they were doing, sitting separately on the buses reserved for the grownups.

On arrival at Cleethorpes the day followed a time-honoured routine. If it wasn't raining we spent what was left of the morning and the early afternoon on the beach. If it rained we spent our time on the slot machines in the arcades on the seafront. The use of the word 'sea' here is not strictly correct. Cleethorpes is on the mouth of the River Humber. The tide would go out so far it used to take sandwiches, and search parties had to be sent out to find it and show it the way back. Around lunchtime, the men all went to the pubs and the women herded large groups of we children together so watching us required less woman-power, and they could take it in turns to slip off and play bingo in the arcades. Mid-afternoon we searched for lost children as some small child always disappeared and was usually found goggle-eyed in front of a particularly brightly lit and/or noisy slot machine of some kind. Then we went to Wonderland, a somewhat exaggerated name for the indoor funfair on the seafront (the chances of finding anything wonderful in Cleethorpes were pretty remote), before leaving at 6 pm prompt.

The regular trips that I make nowadays are to visit the kids. Clare is now a freelance musician in Scotland and is having a whale of a time. She has two websites and is now more than making ends meet. Meanwhile, James is in his second year at Sussex, heavily involved in the Drama Society and is not making ends meet. His financial situation should, fortunately, be improved by the fact that he has recently been banned from all the bars at Sussex University. I can't think where he gets it from. It's all a bit of a storm in a teacup really. He was performing in a play called 'Shit Shakespeare' which required James's half of the cast to be drunk. And they take their art very seriously in Sussex University Drama Society, so he tells me.

I think James's financial situation could be much improved if he got a job in the summer. I worked during the summer vacation, and sometimes during the Christmas holidays, from the ages of 15 to 21. I use the word 'worked' very loosely. For example, I was employed at a frozen food factory one summer, allegedly hosing down the insides of refrigerated lorries but their turn round was usually too quick to allow time for this. And so I spent most of my time doing 'The Sun' crossword with one of my workmates, propping up a brush in the 'garage', making tea for the others, and looking as busy as possible. I spent another summer working on a small building site, where many of my duties were extra-curricular: going to the bar at lunchtimes to fetch drinks while the lads played dominoes, making the tea, fetching the fish and chips on Fridays, and collecting 'surplus' bricks to put in the back of the foreman's van – he was building an extension at home.

I also worked in several factories. At the canning factory the best job was in the warehouse, where you could go and hide at the top of the stacks of boxes of cans. There was a whole world up there, a maze of constantly changing 'rooms' within the boxes, where you could sleep, play cards, open and eat cans of fruit. It wouldn't have surprised me to find a TV, or even a fully stocked bar and discotheque up there. You were out of sight and out of mind, actually out of your mind with boredom, as working with tin cans is not intrinsically rewarding. There's only so much you can do with a can. It doesn't laugh at your jokes and can't play chess. At the chicken factory, the chickens were also unresponsive, although they were mostly dead, and those that weren't, the new arrivals, soon would be. I did, however, learn how to throw a chilled chicken corpse onto a hook from a distance of six feet, a skill I found particularly useful when returning undergraduate essays. Come to think of it, many undergraduates are not unlike the chickens, or indeed, the tin cans or the surplus bricks.

Both James and Clare provide us with regular opportunities to get rid of surplus cash, and to go for short breaks in Glasgow and Brighton to watch them perform in something or other. I quite like both cities and now know good hotels and restaurants in both. Lizzie, our youngest daughter, is the only one living at home and will be completing a part-time Master's at the University of Edgbaston in September next year. We shall be going to her graduation at some stage. She continues to work part-time at Lloyds Bank. Anne is still working part-time at the hospital and will probably not now retire until 2014, if she can stand it that long. She is very much at odds with what seems to be the prevailing NHS philosophy, that nursing is about looking after computers rather than looking after patients. Computers-on-wheels (or COWs, as they are called) can also cause unforeseen problems. Recently, a patient sat waiting for treatment in Casualty was somewhat miffed to hear a doctor ask a nurse to "wheel in the COW from the next cubicle".

Of course, 2012 was a big year for sport and I can't end without making some comment on the London Olympics, which I quite enjoyed. Some of the things they give medals for are amazing. Synchronised diving, for example, why diving? Why not synchronised cycling or juggling or whatever? A particular favourite of mine is shooting, especially small-bore shooting, which for some reason conjures up a rather pleasing image of a five foot tall politician, or estate agent, being pursued by a pack of men with handguns. And isn't it amazing how we all become interested in badminton, cycling, archery, dressage (one of the silliest events imaginable and why only horses? Why not dogs or sheep or hamsters?) and rowing for a few days every four years. It's the complete arbitrariness of what is included and excluded, and who is included and excluded that fascinates me. I'm sure I noticed baseball in there somewhere. Is anyone other than the USA and, presumably Canada, able to send a team? What next? Gaelic Football Ireland versus Northern Ireland? Or bullfighting? Spain A versus… Spain B? And, as I've said already, why are horses welcome but not dogs? And why didn't we introduce sheepdog trials in 2012, we would have at least been certain of getting a bronze medal then, behind Australia and New Zealand, obviously. And what about snooker and darts?

Of course, the other great arbitrary element of the Olympics is that you don't know who is on drugs and who isn't. It used to be easy to work this out, at least retrospectively. For example, if that petite East German or Chinese girl who won a gold medal in gymnastics in one Olympics then grew a beard and went on to win a bronze or silver in the men's wrestling at a subsequent Olympics, you could be pretty certain she was on steroids the first-time round. Conversely, the fact that we British rarely won anything was clear evidence that our athletes weren't taking drugs, or couldn't afford drugs, or were giving them to our horses because drug abuse has now become much more sophisticated and has spread to non-human competitors. At Beijing, four horses were disqualified from the show jumping because they had been given a de-sensitising drug, which deadened the feeling in their legs and encouraged them to lift their feet up more when they were jumping. I kid you not. I bet their riders felt damn silly running around the arena and jumping the fences without a horse underneath them. This conjures up some intriguing questions. Is our countryside populated by Mafia-type gangs of equine drug dealers? Is there a top-horse, presumably called the Godstallion, who warns off his enemies by leaving a man's head in the straw in their stables? And finally, changing the focus, what exactly was Champion the Wonder Horse (of the famous 1960's children's TV series) taking that made him so wonderful? I suppose we will never know.

Turning to football, I am really not so keen on the World Cup. I hate watching the England football team. You know they are always going to eventually lose in the quarter final to Germany or Argentina, probably after a penalty shoot-out. Or lose to some team of nobodies ranked 120 places below them, probably after a penalty shoot-out. Or lose because the manager, who has changed from a hero to a villain in 90 minutes, got the tactics wrong and has been forced to resign, probably after a penalty shoot-out. It is something of a relief when England have been knocked out. You can enjoy the remaining games with no tension. Sometimes I think it is a pity we won WW2, probably after a penalty shoot-out, and wish we had allowed the Germans to win in return for their post-WW2 record in World Cup tournaments.

As I write this on November 26th, Anne tells me the road at the bottom/side of the garden is closed because of flooding further along it. Extreme weather seems to be the norm these days and, so much so that I tend to associate Christmas with heavy rain rather than snow. So, here's hoping for a dry one this year!

Merry Christmas

NOVEMBER 2013

Christmas approaches yet again. This year can hardly be as momentous and chaotic as it was last year. It began with a phone call from Anne to Angie on Christmas Eve, which was answered by our (then) five-year-old granddaughter, who told her mummy couldn't come to the phone because she had 'wet herself'. Angie's waters had broken. To cut a long story short, plans to attend Midnight Mass were abandoned and Angie eventually gave birth to our second grandson, Colin, in the early hours of Christmas Day. It led to a somewhat muted but very happy Christmas Day, which we had to re-run on New Year's Day for Angie's benefit.

The year 2013 was generally a big one for us, as Anne and I had our 60th birthdays, James had his 21st and Anne's dad had his 90th. We celebrated with a family holiday (as you do) in Switzerland. It was a train holiday, 20 train journeys and over 2000 miles travelled, with great weather and magnificent mountain views. Healthwise, I withstood the demands of so much travel very well, although Anne's dad struggled a bit.

Actually, his biggest problem is increasingly his deafness. Allied to my poor speech, this makes communication between us is quite difficult. I can't say what I want to say and he can't hear what I'm saying anyway. This leads to his answers to my questions being based on pure guesswork. For example, I might ask him "Do you want a drink?" and he answers "Twenty to three." But, in general, he is doing very well and we had a big party recently to celebrate his birthday.

Quickly moving on, you may remember last year I commented on the Americans' inability to select presidential candidates with sensible names (that is, other than Mitt and Barack). Well, I've discovered even more silly American names. Sarah Palin, former Alaska governor and vice-presidential candidate, has a son called Track. What sort of a name is that? Is Mrs. Palin completely mad? (Don't answer that.) It could have been worse, I suppose, she might have called him Railing Palin. At the end of last year, Mrs. Palin's kids were apparently having marital difficulties. Track was divorcing his wife, Britta, whilst Palin's daughter, Bristol (it could also have been worse, she might have been called Glastonbury or Shepton Mallet or, even Llanfairpwllgwyngyll-gogerychwyrndrobwllllantysiliogogogoch) had parted from her partner, Levi, who had gone on to marry someone called Sunny. Presumably he found her sisters Rainy, Drizzly and Occasional Showers too wet (alright, I made the last bit up). Come back Bob Geldof and Fifi Trixiebell, and the man who named his son after the entire Liverpool football team, all is forgiven.

In an attempt to get out and about more, I have recently joined UA3 (the University of the Third Age) which has turned out to be a slightly strange experience. UA3 consists of a wide range of groups, over 80 of them in Worcester, which meet fortnightly. I attended my first meeting in late October, the board and card games group, expecting it to be populated mainly by highly competitive men playing highly competitive and aggressive board games. I was quite surprised to find myself with no other men but 11 old ladies, with three of whom I spent the afternoon playing whist. It wasn't an unpleasant experience and I will go again, but it was not exactly what I'd expected.

I've got to decide now which of the other groups I am going to join. There are all the usual ones: local history, genealogy, walking (going for walks), travel (going on trips) and I may well join one or more of these. Then there are the practical ones: computing, various gardening ones and lots of languages, mostly modern but, intriguingly, Latin is also available and I quite fancy it. I'm a great believer in the usefulness of learning Latin. Never mind bringing back National Service for all the yobs in society, get them conjugating Latin verbs and reading Vergil's Aeniad, and they won't have time for all those drugs and tattoos and collecting ASBOs! I did Latin at 'O' Level and found it had three great advantages over modern languages:

1. It had less words for you to learn. 2000 years ago many things were not invented, like stress and TV quiz show panellists, or simply did not exist, like Mars Bars and steamrollers. This makes it much easier to learn the required vocabulary. A Roman soldier would just never say, "Pass me my iPod, Brutus."

2. There was much less history about at the time of the

Roman Empire and so much less to write about. During the two years I studied for Latin 'O' level, most of our readings were about Hannibal crossing the Alps with his elephants, which he did on a fairly regular basis. It was good exciting stuff, if a bit repetitive. None of this "Pierre goes to the *boulangerie* or *la gare* or *l'école*," rubbish that we got in French. Hannibal was a kind of Indiana Jones figure whereas Pierre was just an annoying little twerp.

3. It used less words than modern languages and has some wonderfully economical words. My favourite is the verb *trepidare* which translates as 'to rush about in panic'.

But I did have one problem with Latin, and that was the verb coming at the end of the sentence. This meant that you knew who was doing it, and you knew who or what they were doing it to, but you didn't know what they were going to do until the very last minute. And it wasn't difficult to come up with examples of when that might be important. For example: I you am going to kiss/kill, I the trousers that you are wearing am going to iron (good)/ take off (even better, if the speaker is the opposite sex)/ set fire to (bad)/ nail to the door while you still have them on (even worse). Consequently, I found Latin potentially very tricky and could never really imagine your average Roman soldier or Roman in the street really speaking it. However, it is still very useful to learn Latin though for all kinds of reasons. Actually, UA3 is a good alternative to going to Parkinson's Society meetings, which can be a little dull and occasionally depressing. Holding the meetings in a hospice (I kid you not) is not really a good idea and whereas I enjoyed the talk on Steam Trains in Worcestershire in the 1950s with a slide show, Anne, inexplicably, found it boring.

UA3 is also a potential alternative to my main interest,

watching rugby union. I have had a season ticket at Worcester Warriors for years but 2013/14 is turning into our worst season ever. Apart from our first friendly warm up game back in August, and a drawn game against an obscure French club, we have lost every game so far and are red hot favourites for relegation from the premiership. It is very depressing, so much so that I have taken to watching the crowd rather than the game. Rugby crowds are very interesting and there are at least six types of supporter I have identified over the years:

- The Dinosaur. He was there on the wing when William Webb Ellis first picked up the ball and carried it. I expect he's probably still there waiting for a pass. He knows everything about the game when it was amateur, but nothing since it went professional. He often wears a smart blazer and carries an umbrella. He used to be a common sight on touchlines, marching up and down, staying in line with play, and talking loudly but he has rapidly become an endangered species at the higher levels of the game, since the beginning of the professional era, as his natural habitat has been gradually eroded. Although he still thrives in sanctuaries at some lower level amateur clubs.

- The Escaped Husband. This is the biggest group. Escaped husbands are to be found congregated in herds in the bars before and after the game, often with a son or daughter in tow, desperately trying to minimise the amount of time left in the weekend for decorating and home improvement, gardening, shopping and visiting relatives. This type of fan is knowledgeable about the game and may well have played it in his youth.

- The Oldie. He has been watching the game for a long time. He is definitely pre-Bill Beaumont and can even remember the golden age when Moseley and Coventry used to win matches, and Worcester knew its place in the West Midlands rugby pecking order and did not have ambitions above its station. He often has a deep knowledge of the game and, if prompted, can usually explain every decision the referee takes. He is, without doubt, the best stranger to sit next to at a rugby match.

- The Enthusiast. This type of fan is easy to identify as he will be completely bedecked in the club colours as will his large entourage: wife, five children, dog, rabbit, goldfish, mother-in-law, etc. who inevitably accompany him. He is also very noisy, to the extent that you can often hear him before you see him. He is well-meaning and helpful but if you sit next to him, it is advisable to wear earplugs, preferably attached via a radio to a local station, if possible one broadcasting a commentary of another rugby match, and nod at him a lot.

- The Dogless Man. He dates back to the 1960s and 1970s when he and his now long-deceased dog used to be able to roam freely all around the ground in the days when virtually all rugby grounds were mostly wide-open spaces with few facilities. He continues to attend matches out of habit but is now a sad shrunken figure who, like The Dinosaur, knows little about the modern game or indeed, the game generally. He spent most of his time in the 1960s and 1970s looking for trees for his dog, or looking for his dog amongst the trees. He is prone to get confused during matches and shout "Come Here Rover" instead of "Come on You Warriors" and often thanks the people sitting next to him for helping him call for his dog.

- The Moaner. He complains about everything: the referee, the weather, the pitch, the pasties, but is frequently most critical of his own team. I once sat next to one of these at an away game at Exeter, whom he was allegedly supporting. Everything Exeter did was wrong, the tactics, the kicking, the line-out calls, the colour of the prop's jockstrap. They replaced the winger on our side of the pitch with another player in the second half after he tried to hang himself from the crossbar at half-time. Dozens of Worcester fans supported Exeter in the second half in an attempt to save lives. I nearly asked him why he continued to come to matches as it obviously upset him so much. Why not go car-crash spotting on the motorway on a Saturday afternoon instead? But as he was eight feet tall and obviously an ex-prop forward of the south-western variety, I decided to keep quiet.

So, what of the family? I hear you ask. Well, not really but I'm going to tell you whether you asked or not. As I indicated earlier, Angie now has four kids and has her hands well and truly full. Anne and I can vouch for this as we took the three eldest kids to visit Clare in Glasgow. They are growing up, the eldest started secondary school in September, but they are still very demanding.

Clare is now making a good living as a pianist, teaching, gigging and accompanying a variety of musical groups, choirs and a jazz singer. Lizzie has just completed her part-time Master's at Edgbaston University and is still working at Lloyds Bank, while James is in his final year at Sussex. He is still involved in drama, we are only just back from a trip to Brighton to see a play he wrote and directed. His next play, in February, is 'The Little Shop of Horrors' in which he plays a man-eating plant from outer space! Anne continues to play the much less exciting role of a part-time nurse.

I end this year with two tales of, how can I put this, 'unusual' drivers. First, from the internet in August:

'A blind journalist was given a month's suspended jail sentence and fined 500 euros by a French court on Friday, for driving while drunk and without a license. The owner of the car, who was also drunk, sat next to the blind man when he drove the vehicle. The pair were arrested on a country road in the early hours of July 25th by police, who spotted their car zig-zagging suspiciously and moving at a very low speed.'

Presumably, the blind man's guide dog was in the back seat navigating! It goes on:

'The police were astounded when the 29-year-old driver informed them he was blind. "I really wanted to do it [drive the car]," the blind man told the court, whilst the owner said he saw "a lot of happiness emanating from him" as he drove.'

I wonder if he saw the terror emanating from the other drivers on the road!

I thought that story could never be beaten for driver stupidity, until I saw the following item on the internet in October:

Polish Driver Follows GPS Directions Into Lake.

'A Polish driver who was too sure of his GPS road navigation device, ended up neck-deep in a lake after ignoring road signs warning of a dead-end ahead, Polish police said. A police spokesman added: "His GPS told him to drive straight ahead and he did." The road ran straight downhill into the lake. The driver placed the first call to emergency services while still inside the sinking van. He and two passengers escaped unharmed.'

Well, that's it for another year, and 2013 was quite a good one on balance.

I hope you and yours are well and your Christmas is merry and happy.

Season's greetings and *deus vobiscum* (may your God be with you).

NOVEMBER 2014

Well, here we are again. Those of you who have been keeping up may remember my fascination with American names in general, and names in the Palin family, in particular. Well, Sarah Palin's brood were in the news again in October ,when they got involved in a brawl at a neighbour's house. Track Palin and Todd Palin both threw punches, and Bristol Palin laid out their host, a lady called Korey Klingenmower (yes - that's a real name). Fortunately, police officer Ruth Adolf was there to sort it all out. I would love to have seen the notebook of the police officer who took a list of the names of those present at the time of the incident.

Actually, Ms. Adolf could have been useful in dealing with another Adolph nearer home. A letter quoted in our local paper, in September, tells the story. 'Worcester Cathedral, host of the Three Choirs Festival, is harbouring a racist...[chorister who] ...has been suspended for impersonating Hitler in front of... visiting German singers.' The mind boggles. Imagine the scene in the cathedral. The choir has just completed an Elgar piece when one of the choristers whips off his cassock to reveal a German uniform, complete with swastikas, puts on a false moustache and jackboots down the aisle singing 'Springtime for Hitler'.

Back to reality. The last year has been a fairly busy one with trips to visit offspring in Glasgow and Brighton, two graduations, two weeks in the Scillies and a day at the Edinburgh Fringe. The last of these was amazing. Edinburgh was very crowded and exciting. Some of the sights were incredible. I can't really believe I saw a man halfway up a free-standing ladder, that is, not propped up against anything. He was dressed in only his underpants, juggling machetes. But I did!

TV presenters have it easy. Imagine if Jeremy Paxman had to spin plates whilst asking the questions on 'University Challenge' or if Graham Norton had to wrestle a bear whilst interviewing guests on his show. They wouldn't be so smug then!

Returning to our Edinburgh trip, we were ostensibly there to see two of our kids perform: James in a comedy review show with friends from Sussex University, and Clare as an accompanying pianist in a concert at St. Giles Cathedral. Both were pretty good and quite well attended.

Turning to the two graduations, these contrasted sharply. Sussex, where James got his BA, was quite informal, typified by the video shown with a jokey welcome from the Chancellor, who is a well-known comic actor. So well known, his name escapes me. There was a gigantic reception afterwards with free wine. James was, as usual, very laid back. For example, only buying the shirt he wore on his way to our hotel, where he got changed for the ceremony. The second graduation, where we celebrated Lizzie's completion of a part-time Master's degree at Edgbaston, was much more formal. I must confess that, despite working for over thirty years at the university, I never attended a degree ceremony, and so it was a new experience for me. I haven't missed much. It strikes me that the whole thing would be much more fun if the academic staff wore fancy dress instead of academic gowns. It would be unforgettable if you received your degree whilst Coco the Clown, Jack the Ripper, Prince Charles, a Dalek and a Worcester chorister dressed as Hitler looked on and applauded.

Rather disappointingly, I have subsequently learnt that as part of the university's 'make life as miserable as possible for the academics' programme, it is now compulsory for lecturers in my old department to attend at least one ceremony every three years. I visited the old place when I went to the graduation and found I now only really know one secretary, the head of department and Mad Rab, the Scotsman, whom you may remember from earlier letters. The good, the bad and the ugly. Mad Rab is now a reformed man, he's finally been ground down by the university system and voted 'no' in the referendum on Scottish independence. The university have treated him very badly over the years. He is a loyal, hardworking, junior lecturer who really cares about his students and deserves much better. I'm glad I left when I did.

On a happier note, we managed a mid-September two-week holiday on the Scillies. We were a bit restricted because I don't walk long distances anymore. But the weather was mostly good and I was able to get on the boats and visit all the smaller islands.

My love affair with islands began with three visits to the Isle of Wight in my late teens. The first two were to the annual camps of the Church Lads Brigade – a kind of Church of England Scouts, and the third was my first ever holiday with friends rather than family. The village Church Lads Brigade company was part of the Doncaster Battalion, which was in turn, part of the Sheffield Regiment. The Church Lads Brigade was run very much on military lines. We did not start punch ups with the local Catholics, but lost no opportunity to go on parade and march about a bit in the village (often), Doncaster (occasionally) and Sheffield (annually). We had uniforms and ranks, I eventually became a sergeant, and drilled a lot, usually in the church hall. We also did much more than this and played a great deal of table-tennis and football especially with our friends from the nearby Bentley company, as well as at the annual Sheffield regiment camp on the Isle of Wight.

I can still remember how exciting I found those early visits to the Church Lads Brigade camp. It began with a journey on a specially chartered train, which ran through the night from Sheffield to Portsmouth. This was followed by a short ferry ride, before arriving on the island early on Saturday morning. Those of us lucky enough to be chosen as bag handlers then had an exhilarating ride on the back of open lorries with the suitcases. Health and safety regulations would never allow such innocent pleasure today. We arrived at the campsite near Bembridge in time for lunch. We were free to do whatever we liked after lunch each day, and so I saw much of the island. However, places we did not get to were the (in?)famous first, in 1969, and second, in 1970, Isle of Wight music festivals, which coincided with the camps. I feel really frustrated that I didn't get to the festivals when I was so close to them. The nearest we got was seeing the large number of hippies who came over on the same ferry as us. The Church Lads Brigade and the Isle of Wight festival audience were not really compatible.

I have been back to the island four times since these early visits. There was a day trip from Bristol, a holiday with my wife, a family holiday, and I hitchhiked there and slept rough for two nights when I was an undergraduate. I would have gone more often but Anne does not care much for the Isle of Wight and finds it too commercialised. I still quite like it and find the commercialised parts, such as the model village at Godshill and the waxworks at Brading, the best bits.

The Scilly Isles are a quite different proposition and have Anne's approval. I have lost count of the number of times we have stayed there, but it must be well into double figures. There are five currently inhabited islands and one that used to be, and you can visit them all by boat. The only other form of transport available is the bicycle; tourists are not allowed to take their cars and there is virtually nowhere to drive to anyway. The Scilly Isles are completely uncommercialised, and in good weather it is close to paradise with wonderful walks and virtually empty beaches. You are a bit dependent on the weather but it is usually good, and you are not disappointed. Above all you are guaranteed to have a relaxed and stress-free holiday. The pace of life is slower on the Scillies somehow.

Turning to the domestic front, Anne and I are finally home alone as Lizzie has now moved out, and lives with her boyfriend on the other side of the town centre. Clare is still in Glasgow and recently played piano for Alex Salmond twice, at an Edinburgh Tattoo dinner, and at a thank you party for those who helped him campaign for Scottish independence. It's a good job he didn't see the 'No' badge in her handbag! She still hasn't met anyone really famous though, like Buffin, Mott the Hoople's drummer, whom I met in 1972. Until recently, I still had the drumstick to prove it.

James recently took part in one of several ads for an employment agency, which, if chosen, will hit your TV screens and/or the internet next year. Angie continues to bring up her two boys (12 and 1, mostly good) and two girls (8 and 7, mostly bad, always fighting each other). Anne's Dad, aged 91, has just had a knee replacement and is currently convalescing with us for a fortnight.

I seem to spend much of my time reading, especially books of the detective whodunnit variety. I particularly like the quirky stuff such as McCall Smith's Botswana-based 'First Ladies' Detective Agency' series and also two seriously weird sets of stories. One is based on a Humphrey Bogart-type detective, set in a kind of sleazy 1930s Aberystwyth, of all places, where the streets are run by gangster-druids. The other, weirdest of all, is about a detective who actually goes inside books and makes sure the characters behave themselves. It's the 'Bookworld' series and is virtually impossible to describe. Arthur Conan Doyle has a lot to answer for. On the basis that even some of the weird stuff gets published, I'm thinking of writing a novel about a detective with a long white beard, who always dresses in red and has a sidekick called Rudolph. I can't think of a name for him though.

And the really big news of 2014 is that Anne retired at the end of June and is now, predictably, busier than she ever was when she had a job. She misses seeing her colleagues but will happily live without getting up at 6 am in January and February, before driving through the early morning rush hour to try and park in the hospital carpark. At the end she had very mixed feelings about retiring as, indeed, did I.

My predominant feeling was a huge sense of relief, tinged with great sadness. I loved my job, although the profession was becoming something of a treadmill towards the end, with a great deal of jumping through hoops and leaving of paper trails. The fun was being sucked out of the job. But as a professor, I was able to rise above the bureaucratic pettiness and still get much pleasure out of the work. It was a job which allowed you to decide your own work programme and hours, and where the only fixed time commitments you faced were your teaching and student contact hours per week and exam meetings in June. I chose a whole range of additional activities, some of which gave me extra income. The most important activity, which gave no extra income, was my involvement with my professional association, the University Association for Contemporary European Studies (UACES), of which I was the treasurer for three years between 1995 and 1997. In addition to signing the cheques and attending monthly meetings in London, I was heavily involved in organising UACES conferences.

Outside my normal teaching, I also ran a number of different courses. I did various paid lectures, for example, on enlargement of the EU to NATO officers at the Royal Military Academy in Greenwich, and a lecture on the EU budget to Chinese local government officers based at the university at Worcester. There were also a number of one-off courses. The first of these involved seven Turks, whom I only found out were coming two days before the start of the academic year. They were supposed to be doing our Master's degree and specialise in EU Studies but, unfortunately, on meeting them I discovered they didn't speak English! However, I saw that as a mere detail, and quickly put together a new combined Diploma in English Language and EU Studies. It involved our English Language for Overseas Students Unit, who jumped on board when I offered them money, and a special course on the EU, for 'special' read 'simple', taught by me. At the other end of the scale we ran a ten-week course for 25 ANC members who were likely to become ambassadors and diplomats. This involved six of us, plus a whole range of visiting speakers, and a two-week field trip to Brussels, Luxembourg and Paris. It involved lots of work and the reward was not only financial; when Nelson Mandela came to the UK we were given front row seats for his speech at Birmingham. I was literally sat within ten feet of the great man.

I also ran two sets of regular courses. For ten years, after my return from local government in 1986, and in cooperation with our Institute for Local Government Studies, I ran short courses for local government officers and councilors on the EU, especially EU grants and loans. But the most lucrative courses were those I ran in the Foreign Office, typically for diplomats between postings. They had normally just completed a period in a country outside of Europe and were about to embark on a posting in an EU member state. These courses paid for the family holiday for nine years in the 1990s.

The most badly paid teaching were the irregular lectures I gave over the years for Extra Mural Studies. I actually put on a whole course one year at a school in a village quite close to Worcester. The one road into this village was prone to flooding, which meant getting to the class was sometimes a bit of a lottery. However, it was a good group and a good course, and my credibility was high after most of them heard me briefly interviewed on Radio 4's 'Today' programme when the EU held a summit meeting at Birmingham in 1992.

It is true that you worked, and I certainly did work, an average of well over 40 hours each week, but you had a lot of control over the content, timing and location of your work. It was a bit like being self-employed. Looking back, I don't know how I fitted it all in. On top of my normal duties, I used to have one or two meetings in London each month, went to Brussels at least once a year, America every other year for a biannual conference, as well as speaking at one-off conferences in the UK and abroad, in China, New Zealand, Israel and Malta. I have to admit that much of the time spent on these activities was at the expense of spending time with my family, which I justified to myself as being necessary to get promoted and/or as a means of increasing our income.

With my PD getting gradually worse, I could not keep up this level of activity, and I increasingly adopted an Edgbaston-first policy in the 2000-2010 period. This meant I gave my commitments at Edgbaston priority. It became progressively more difficult to do even this, and much of the relief I felt on retiring came from not having to continually hold myself together and keep up the appearance of normality. On retirement, I was able to relax, let things go and not continuously fight my PD. This is why, I believe, I went so rapidly downhill in the period from October 2010 to 2011, and probably why so many people fade away quickly and even die soon after retirement.

But it's all history now.

So, let me wish you a Merry Christmas and a Happy New Year!

NOVEMBER 2015

Wasn't the election exciting? I found the contrast between the looks and personalities of the party leaders quite fascinating. Cameron and Miliband, the dashing head prefect and the ugly duckling, fresh-faced choir boy, with Farage as the school bully and Clegg as his victim. In truth, Clegg was more like Father Dougal to Cameron's Father Ted, and I swear Farage is a direct descendant of the spiv, Private Walker, in Dad's Army. Ultimately, while I enjoyed the election campaign, I found the results disturbing. I cannot understand how we can continue with a First Past The Post voting system that generates such unrepresentative results, although I'm not sure what we should replace it with.

Just like the election results, Scotland tends to rather dominate my letter this year. As if visiting our daughter in Glasgow regularly wasn't enough, we went to Scotland for a ten-day holiday in late May. The weather was mostly terrible, rainy, windy and cold. Well, mostly Scottish I suppose. We started and finished in Edinburgh, which has become a kind of

Scottish Disneyland, stayed in hotels near Fort William and in Inverness, with very brief visits to Mull and Skye.

Two words of warning. First, take my advice. Do not go to Glencoe, there is nothing there except a very cold, strong wind. There was a massacre there, they had to do something to pass the time, but it was years ago and we already know who did it and all the bodies are gone. All there is to see is a tacky 'museum', with several very small rooms with doors so low you have to virtually belly dance your way through them. Second, be wary of Scottish castles. At least the two that we saw. The reason they are so well preserved is that each castle has been rebuilt and is probably no older than your house. The castles are there to confuse Americans. As I said, we did visit two islands – for half an hour each. We had a bowl of soup in a howling gale on Mull, and half-hour bus tour to nowhere on Skye while the driver gave a commentary in the style of one of the Marx brothers. Unfortunately Harpo, the silent one, rather than Groucho, the wise-cracking one. Actually, we travelled more by train than coach; this was after all, a Great Rail Holiday.

Unfortunately, I went down with a chest infection which required two visits to a doctor. On the second visit I was advised I 'probably ought to be in hospital' but I didn't fancy it much, certainly not in Inverness! We had taken the precaution of going on holiday with a couple, of which the male half was a doctor, but a paediatrician wasn't much use to me. It probably looks as though the holiday was something of a disaster, but on balance the good points outweighed the bad and, in a harsh sort of way, it was bizarrely enjoyable. The scenery and lochs/lakes were fantastic and the train rides, especially on the steam train that went over the viaduct in the

Harry Potter films, were good as were the company and the hotels. Edinburgh and Inverness are well worth a visit, and we did get to sample some haggis.

We were in Edinburgh again at the end of August to see James and Clare perform in the Fringe. We also managed to take in a couple of other shows this year, as well as the usual street performers. There was no man in underpants this time but there was some machete juggling in the streets. Clare has just moved from Glasgow to Edinburgh and so we stayed in her flat for part of the time. Lizzie plus boyfriend also came for a few days.

On the PD front, the local PD Society has reinvented itself as the joint Malvern-Worcester branch and now meets at a much better time and place. To be specific, the play area of one of those new granny villages, where the over-55s can live in sheltered accommodation and play bingo every night. In truth, I quite like the place as it has, in reverse order of interest, a coffee shop, library and bar. I'm not sure they've got the content of the meetings quite right yet as the first event was a talk on local polecats, with some reference to weasels and ferrets. It was well up there with 'steam trains in Worcester in the 1950s' (see earlier letter) but I don't see why it was thought that people with Parkinson's would be particularly interested in ferrets and polecats. Cats perhaps, but no more interest in polecats than in pole vaulting or pole dancing. Now there's a thought, an illustrated talk on pole-dancing...

I had a day in hospital in July, having the battery that powers my deep brain stimulation replaced. I had to be at the QE in Edgbaston by 7 am and the 20-minute operation was over by 9 am. It was all rather dull. I think all the interesting patients were still asleep. It's a pity Anne wasn't asleep in the supermarket later on when, in response to the question "Which apples do you want?" she said loudly "I like Cox". Two old ladies nearby nearly fell over.

It is now 20 years since I was diagnosed with Parkinson's Disease and the future is not too promising. Parkinson's is a degenerative disease and is therefore only likely to get worse. A cure will be found but exactly when depends on the money spent on research into the disease and at least three other factors:

- Firstly, luck. It is quite possible the breakthrough will come by accident, perhaps even as a side effect of something totally unconnected to PD.
- Secondly, a more effective treatment (a new drug?) may be found which falls short of an actual cure, but which revolutionises the treatment of PD.
- Thirdly, the search for a cure may be held back by the controversy surrounding gene research.

In the light of all this, I think the likelihood of my being given some cure for PD in the future is small. PD will continue to play the bridesmaid to dementia and Alzheimer's bride in brain research funding and, even if a cure for PD is found in my lifetime, I will be considered too old to be worth treating. In terms of PD-free years of life added, it is much more cost-effective to treat younger people with PD, hence the older I get the lower I am in the list of priorities. Consequently, I pin my hopes on the development of new treatments, and my prayers for a huge slice of luck. So, it's basically more of the same in the future. I shall simply keep making do with what I've got and taking the drugs. We are all dealt different cards in life and can only play the ones we've got. It's no good complaining, you have to be practical.

Enough of the heavy stuff. On the domestic front, one of the joys (?) of retirement is that you spend more time babysitting your grandchildren. To this end, I found myself sat listening as my 9 year old granddaughter read from a book of nursery rhymes last week. Have you ever thought about the content of these rhymes? It includes homelessness and child abuse – the old woman who lived in a shoe with her kids who she whipped soundly and sent them to bed. There's cruelty to animals and knife crime ('she cut off their tales with a carving knife' and 'ding dong bell, pussy's in the well'), abuse of the mentally ill (Simple Simon) and what do we make of 'Yankee Doodle came to town, riding on a pony; he stuck a feather in his cap, and called it macaroni'. Who is this lunatic sat on a horse in the shopping precinct, pointing at a feather in his hair and shouting "Macaroni"? "Oh don't worry, its only Mr. Doodle, he can go over there and wait with Doctor Foster in the puddle, or the Grand Old Duke of York on the hill until the men in white coats come to take them away." The mind boggles.

Turning to the family, the girls are relatively settled. Angie has her hands full with four kids. In particular, her youngest daughter fills up an arm and a leg all by herself, but she copes well. Clare is making a decent living as a musician, now based in Edinburgh, whilst Lizzie is living happily with her boyfriend and newly-acquired kitten just on the other side of town. James, though, doesn't know what he wants to do. He is now back living at home, having been brought back from Brighton in an epic journey, involving a rare drive outside Worcester for Anne and me playing the role of navigator. It was not easy finding a route that involved no motorways, nor 'fast' dual carriageways, and not getting lost on obscure B-roads. I now understand why Captain Oates walked to his death rather than continue with Scott of the Antarctic. Scott was probably insisting on a route to the South Pole that involved no snow or ice, and drove Oates mad. They should probably have shot Scott and not the huskies when they ran out of food.

I end on a philosophical note this year with some questions for you to contemplate over the holiday period.

Who was Sammy Davis senior?

Why do we tip taxi and coach drivers but not train and bus drivers?

Why didn't Joseph book a hotel room in advance, particularly as they were travelling during the Christmas period?

What if the Hokey Cokey really is what it's all about?

Think about it.

In the unlikely event that you have any answers to these queries, please include them with the next Christmas card that you send us.

Merry Christmas.

NOVEMBER 2016

Here we are again. Christmas Day was very different for us last year. It was a much quieter affair, which we hope to repeat this year, with only five of us instead of the usual 13 or 14 for dinner. Angie decided her kids had reached the stage where they didn't want to go visiting on Christmas Day. While it may be true to say we missed the pitter-patter of tiny feet, we didn't miss the running, shouting, screaming, crying and fighting of Anne as the cooking of a meal for 14 finally drove her over the edge. The family still all came to us on Boxing Day.

It has not really been the best of years for me as I have not been too well. In particular, my speech is quite bad. I have developed the typical Parkinson's quiet voice and have a bit of a stutter. Consequently, I find talking difficult sometimes, although many would say that this is a good thing! Also, I don't walk well and need a wheelchair for longer distances. I actually fell over in the hydrotherapy pool a few weeks ago and the physiotherapist jumped in, fully clothed, to rescue me. I think she over-reacted, though having someone die in your class probably involves a lot of paperwork. At any rate, I have had to abandon my plans to swim the Channel, given up clog and tap dancing (I kept falling off anyway) and I have informed the England football team manager I am not available for the rest of the season.

I'm very lucky really in that I've had little in the way of side effects from taking my drugs. The NHS is big on these and likes to provide an extensive list ranging from 'feeling drowsy' to 'growing lots of facial hair and calling yourself Mr. Hyde'. The last of these is a particular worry to women, and to men sat next to women in doctors' surgeries. Indeed, taking the drugs can turn you into a compulsive gambler or sex addict. Quite a few older ladies have been very surprised by the reawakening of their husband's interest in 'bedtime activities' and I'm sure it featured in a divorce case somewhere a few years ago. "I admit I committed adultery once, your honour, with the Wimbledon ladies' netball team, but the incident with the lady bishop on the train was due to me mishearing her because of my deafness, I thought she said 'Let us play.'"

My poor health has meant we haven't done much this year. We did manage an extended trip to Edinburgh during the Fringe where we saw Clare and James perform, on the same day actually. Clare's concert was a very straight classical recital in a cathedral with an audience of 100 + and contrasted sharply with James's sketch show. We wondered where he was at the beginning and why he told us not to sit on the front row. However, both questions were answered when he appeared at the back and ran through the audience to the stage wearing nothing but a pair of tartan underpants, with a banana inside them which he proceeded to peel and eat! Our travels were also constrained by Anne having to make several extended visits to Bristol to see her Dad who, at the age of 92, came back from Spain with Legionnaires Disease. He was very ill in hospital for some time but is now fully recovered, and spent his 93rd birthday in Belgium, which is suitably quiet. I've spent more time in Belgium, particularly Brussels, than I would have liked. Brussels is actually quite dull. Once you've seen the Grande Place there isn't much there except a creaky, old remnant of the 1958 World Trade Fair (the Atomium) and the beers and the bars. Whenever I have gone there it has always been wet and cold and there seems to be scaffolding everywhere. I suppose a scaffolder wearing a raincoat, with a taste for beer and the 1950s, might like it but I prefer Bruges, and even Ghent has its attractions.

It is probably true to say that Anne and I seem to spend much of our time in Malvern. My hydrotherapy and speech therapy classes are held there, and for a while I went to yoga classes as well. I can't say I was much taken by yoga. It always seems like exercise for the slow and lazy to me, although I admit that I may be missing something here. We were also part of a small group of PD sufferers taken up to the summit of the Malvern Hills in Land Rovers, and got our picture in the local paper. As, indeed, did James when he organised an open mic comedy night in October. Anne likes Malvern so much, she would like to live there but I have doubts about moving somewhere where the high street is so steep you need mountaineering equipment to get up it. And which Malvern do you live in? There are at least five, all quite different: Malvern Link, Great Malvern, West Malvern, Malvern Wells and Little Malvern. It is very confusing.

We lived in Sheffield when I took unpaid leave of absence and worked for South Yorkshire County Council (SYCC) from 1983 until 1985. My job consisted of providing information about the EU, EU lobbying activities and applying for EU grants and loans. I applied for millions of pounds. I was also working in a quite different environment, with flexi-time, an open plan office and travel to work as part of a carpool. (The office was in Barnsley but I lived in Sheffield.) I adapted surprisingly well and enjoyed it tremendously. There were about ten of us in the office, with Economic Services the smaller of two departments. There were technically five of us in Economics, although one effectively worked elsewhere, and one was a Sheffield city councilor. I can honestly say that during my time with SYCC I saw him more times on the local television news than I did in the office.

Nor were the local 'celebrities' with links to the office restricted to him. Geoffrey Boycott lived next door to one colleague, and David Blunkett lived around the corner from me. I used to see him with his kids in the children's room of one of the local pubs most Sunday lunchtimes. I lived in Grenoside, a suburb on the northern tip of Sheffield. It was virtually a separate village and living there had very much a village feel to it, with massive woods nearby and the Peak District national park only 4 miles away. It also had a full range of village shops, an annual running race, the Grenoside Chase, which passed in front of our house. Morris dancers performed outside a local pub, only yards from our front door, every Boxing Day. We loved it and were very sorry to leave; it puts Malvern in the shade.

Changing the subject, I actually spent much of this year following the EU debate and did, eventually, join in in a small way by having two letters published in the local paper. The second of these was a reaction to our local MP's views on Brexit. He's called Robin but ought to be called Turkey because his desire to welcome Britain leaving the EU is not dissimilar to a Turkey looking forward to Christmas. Apologies to any Brexit supporters reading this. But turning to the referendum, I found the whole debate embarrassing. The Brexit side set the level very low by basing their campaign on the £350 million NHS lie, and outrageously refused to admit it was a lie. Politicians have no shame or honour at all anymore, and have now joined the ranks of bankers, estate agents and solicitors, that is, people who can legally rip you off, in my mind. Then the Remain side, instead of sticking to the high ground, joined Brexit in the gutter – and so it went on. The Brexit supporters did not know, quite literally, what they were voting for and it quickly became clear that different parts of Brexit were voting for different things. Little attention was paid to the wider and indirect implications of the outcome. For example, the debate will almost certainly trigger another Scottish independence referendum which will probably vote 'yes', leaving the Labour Party, which relies on seats in Scotland, permanently out of power in Conservative England. Finally, many Brexit supporters appeared to believe that a departing UK could simply take a shopping list to Brussels and just tick off what it wanted, Unfortunately the world doesn't work like that

I also followed the American presidential debate with interest. Could the Democrats really not have found a better candidate than Honest Emailing Hillary? The result did not surprise me. The Americans are very insular and many of them don't even have passports, so policies like the Mexican wall and protectionism play well there. James held a similar view and placed a small bet on a Trump victory, and won £50! This tendency towards insularity is aggravated by Trump's ignorance about foreign policy. Let's hope Trump learns quickly because before the election the only things that could be said in his favour were he has a sensible first name and the search for the next James Bond villain was over: Trump is perfect. That's probably enough politics. Trump is too easy a target and I'm beginning to sound like the mild-mannered, Maltese taxi driver when I spoke at a conference there some years ago and said, as we passed through one of the (rare) isolated parts: "I could sort out all Malta's political problems in a few minutes if I could bring a machine gun and 20 politicians of my choice out here," or words to that effect. I was the external examiner of a Maltese student's PhD thesis a few years earlier, I'm glad I passed him.

Finally. I return to Christmas, with a list of Christmas cracker jokes:

Why is Santa so jolly?
Because he knows where all the naughty girls live.

What did Adam say to his wife at Christmas?
It's Christmas, Eve!

What do you call people who are afraid of Santa Claus?
Claustrophobic.

What does Santa bring naughty boys and girls on Christmas Eve?
A pack of batteries with a note saying 'toy not included'.

What do get if you cross a duck and Santa.
A Christmas quacker.

What's the difference between snowmen and snowladies ?
Snowballs.

What do you get when you cross a snowman with a vampire?
Frostbite.

Which Christmas carol is a favorite of parents?
Silent Night.

How many reindeer does it take to change a light bulb?
Eight. One to screw in the light bulb and seven to hold
Rudolph down.

What do you call a blind reindeer?
I have no eye deer.

What do you call a singing elf with sideburns?
Elfis.

What do you call an elf wearing ear muffs?
Anything you want. He can't hear you.

What goes "Oh oh oh"?
Santa walking backwards.

What do you call a bunch of chess players bragging about their
games in a hotel lobby?
Chess nuts boasting in an open foyer.

Who delivers Christmas presents to dogs?
Santa paws.

Who delivers Christmas presents to cats?
Santa claws.

What did Santa Claus say to his wife about the weather?
It's going to reindeer.

And I end with another question to which I've always wanted to know the answer:

Why doesn't Tarzan have a beard?

Merry Christmas.

NOVEMBER 2017

Last year's Christmas got off to a cracking start. Those of you who have had the luck, not sure if it's good or bad, to have shared a flat with me (or visited such a flat) will be aware of my great liking for a certain Jethro Tull, led by flautist Ian Anderson. I've seen them over 20 times and nowadays don't listen much to anyone else. This is not as repetitive as it may initially seem, given their 60 or so albums of various kinds, plus loads of stuff on the internet, around 400 songs in total, many of them in multiple versions. Now, Anderson and Friends, as I think they are usually billed, have taken to playing charity Christmas concerts at cathedrals, and last year played Worcester. It gets even better because on the way back to our seats at the interval, who should we bump into on his way back to the stage but the great man himself, with whom we exchanged a few words. And very pleasant he was too!

Christmas wasn't half-bad either and the presents were quite good, although I'm not sure that my giving Anne the complete Leonard Cohen studio albums was such a good idea. Life is depressing enough without listening to Cohen, who is now not so much depressed as deceased. She countered with a book, supposedly written by Enid Blyton, entitled 'Five on Brexit Island' with lashings of wit, irony and sarcasm! However, I felt that 2016, in general, and Christmas, in particular, were somewhat marred by the number of celebrity deaths, which seemed to turn into an avalanche as the end of the year approached. Some big names died in 2016. I can probably live without Cilla Black and Val Doonican, but Bowie, Prince, Muhammad Ali, Victoria Wood, Alan Rickman, Gene Wilder and Arnold Palmer, what a team for a rugby sevens tournament! And then, after Greg Lake in early- and Zsa Zsa Gabor in mid-December, there was a surge with Rick Parfitt (Status Quo), George Michael, Debbie Reynolds and her daughter Carrie Fisher all departing in quick succession in late December. Perhaps a set of Leonard Cohen CDs was rather a good choice of gift, after all. He also died in 2016 but I didn't include him earlier as part of the sevens team because he has a tendency to get over-excited and keep shouting "Hallelujah!"

On balance though, 2017 hasn't been a good year. In May, Clare got food poisoning from supermarket chicken, we think, and was very ill. Weeks went by and she wasn't getting any better, and her GP eventually gave her two different antibiotics but did nothing else, although she was losing weight. Finally, she saw another GP who sent her straight to hospital. After various attempts to treat her medically, her consultant said, "You are significantly sick and need surgery urgently." They operated immediately and, thankfully, it did the trick. Anne was in Edinburgh for nearly three weeks but Clare recovered well and was fit enough to play the piano for two hours non-stop, there was no interval, for a production of 'Sweeney Todd' at the Edinburgh Fringe. Then it was my turn, when I had yet another spell in Worcester hospital in October 2017. It all began shortly before a trip to Yorkshire, visiting my sister and breaking the world record for most relatives visited in two days, when I fell over on the drive and banged my back. I had a chest infection at the time and went to the doctor, who sent me to hospital to have a chest X-ray, and as an afterthought to have my back X-rayed.

I went to Yorkshire and back, and got on with life only to discover eventually that my chest wasn't too bad but I'd fractured a vertebra in my back. My GP sent me straight back to A&E for more X-rays, specifically to check no bits of bone had got into the spinal canal. I was lucky – they hadn't. I spent nine hours on a trolley in a corridor in A&E, before they eventually decided I needed bed rest and admitted me at 1 am. I spent 14 of the most boring and weird days of my life as I lived in my bed, not allowed to even walk to the toilet. I thought I was never going to get out. For several days I experienced vivid dreams, nightmares and hallucinations. I kept waking up in an extended version of our cubicle, which had become one of those houses of horrors you used to find at fairs. I longed to get out of bed and investigate but could not move because of my Parkinson's.

However, I could make threats and, at one point, I remember I came out with the following: "I've got a gun and I'm going to shoot the next person who comes in through the window." Now, I'm not sure whether I merely thought this or actually said it. I could have sworn the nurse who brought me breakfast the following day was wearing a bullet-proof vest under her uniform. Anyway, I was not at my best and was glad to get home a few days later. That's the second time I've left hospital feeling much worse than I went in and I'm beginning to have doubts about the NHS.

Matters were not helped by the fact that I was also plagued yet again by old men shouting through the night. One of them was prone to shout about shutting the latch to keep Betty in and the animals out, whilst another thought he was being chased by someone called Albert or Arthur. I tried to reassure them but unfortunately, my attempts to talk to other patients in their sleep were a complete failure and we returned to the unlatched door, Betty and Albert/Arthur on several subsequent occasions. It really was like a mad house in there. Back in the real world, I was talking nonsense, I was confused and didn't know where I was. I continued with this recurring nightmare for the best part of a week. Anne was convinced all of this was due to me being excessively dehydrated. I was eventually sent home, and I have to wear a back brace at least until I see the consultant in late December/early January. I feel like a snail dragging my shell around and I'm bracing myself for Christmas (BOOM! BOOM!). However, the biggest problem is not being able to take a shower. Instead, Anne has to use her nursing skills and give me a bed bath daily, as I'm not allowed out of bed until the brace is on. This is okay but she does get a bit fed up of wearing the uniform.

Fortunately, my lack of mobility is not the big problem that it might have been with Christmas approaching. I now buy most of my Christmas presents online, partly because I have grown to hate conventional shopping over the years. I blame Anne for this. She is the most frustrating shopper ever. I will happily go out to buy a pair of shoes and, if I am in the right mood, will return two hours later with a jacket, four shirts and two pairs of trousers. Anne, on the other hand, will go shopping for five hours and return with a salad and a cardigan, which she will take back the following day because she's decided she can't eat one and the other is too big for her. I'm not sure which is which. If you cannot avoid shopping with your wife, I find following a few basic principles essential:

- Never follow your wife around the shop. Remain at the point where she starts to look at things. SHE WILL ALWAYS RETURN TO WHERE SHE STARTED. You can save yourself a great deal of energy if you follow this principle.

- Take a book and some sandwiches, and know where the chairs are in Marks & Spencer's. You are going to spend a lot of time there. In fact, during the sales it is as well to take a small tent and a sleeping bag.

- Know the nearest pub to her favourite shops. Thus, for example, when the kids were young I used to know how to get from Mothercare or the Early Learning Centre to the nearest pub within six minutes in at least five city centres. If you are really lucky, you might be able to convince her that, as you always rush her, it is better if you leave her in peace. In this case, by going to the pub, you are actually doing her a favour. This is the marriage equivalent of scoring 180 in darts or making a maximum break in snooker!

- Be ready to sympathise with her because THEY WILL NEVER HAVE WHATEVER SHE WANTS IN HER SIZE.

I cannot go any further without commenting on the big news of the year. A new Doctor Who was announced recently and it is a woman. I have nothing against this in principle and, indeed, welcome the addition of strong female characters, such as Ace – she of the baseball-beating dalek fame – to the programme. But, the Doctor becoming a woman does raise a number of problems. Most obviously, how the new Doctor will cope with the shock of going to the toilet for the first time and discovering that not every part of his/her body has successfully regenerated. Also, as the Doctor started kissing girlies, something to which I wholeheartedly object, in his eighth reincarnation, where does becoming a woman leave him/her sexually-speaking? Is the new Doctor Who a new category of transsexual or is she a perverted lesbian who likes men? It is all very confusing, and it is not until we have seen the new Doctor in action and fans have started to put her in their rankings of Doctor Whos that it will be possible to answer these questions. My own favourite Doctor Who is the unfashionable Sylvester McCoy (Doctor number 7) followed by Troughton (2) with Tom Baker (4), Tennant (10) and Smith (11) fighting out the next three places. The rest are either joint sixth – Hartnell (1), Pertwee (3), Davison (5) and Capaldi (12) – or were not in the role long enough to be assessed – Colin Baker (6), McGann (8) and Eccleston (9). McCoy too was not given enough time. He only appeared in three short series, but each one built and improved on the previous one, and his series four and five would have been very good indeed had they been made.

Changing, the subject, I have now completed 22 years of having Parkinson's Disease and I have been reflecting on the early years. One thing that does surprise me retrospectively is that no-one ever talked to me about my Parkinson's at work. No-one asked me how I was when I went in or showed any curiosity about PD and asked me questions. It was almost as if it was a taboo subject, which it was not as far as I was concerned, or perhaps they just didn't care, or know, that I had PD. Perhaps it was me who failed to talk to them about it. To be fair, I didn't go to any social staff occasions and the department did have a high turnover of staff at this time. Many of the more longstanding staff, including most of the colleagues that I'd known for years, moved to other universities and I didn't mix much with the newer members of staff because I rarely saw them. The department was a cold, empty place and I must have been something of a mystery man to the newer members of staff, and certainly would have been to the students. However, I am still surprised that the head of department or head of school didn't take me to one side from time to time and ask me how things were going.

Turning finally to the family. Anne has been retired several years now but is replacing her job with the role of carer for me and, increasingly, for the grandkids, as Angie is in the process of splitting up with her partner. Anne's Dad is still going strong at the age of 94. Having recovered from Legionnaire's Disease, he has just returned from a holiday at the same hotel where he became ill. Meanwhile, Lizzie has a new job at a small local theatre/arts centre. This is the sort of work she wants to do and so she is much happier than she was at Lloyds. James has got a job in an office and continues with his drama/comedy. He did the Edinburgh Fringe and runs a monthly stand-up comedy night at a local pub in Worcester. He has also done some stand-up himself at pubs in Edgbaston and finally seems to be sorting himself out. We've got no idea what precisely he does in his office, but as far as we can tell it is perfectly legal and doesn't involve killing anyone, and so we are quite happy with it. They keep sending him to their HQ at Swindon for training and putting him up (all expenses paid) at a hotel, which is a new experience for him. It's quite amazing how much difference having a job makes.

I remember getting my job at Edgbaston. Warwick was a

good place from which to apply for a job. I actually received two offers, the other one being from North London Polytechnic. In fact, I initially accepted the London job but pulled out when I was interviewed for and got the job at Edgbaston, on the advice of my PhD supervisor who told me to "go for the proper university". My first interview had been at East Anglia in Norwich, a ridiculous affair with a panel of 14 for what was a junior lectureship. I sometimes reflect on how life consists of a number of crossroads at which you take key decisions. I could have easily ended up in Norwich, London, Plymouth or Swansea and had a completely different life. My job title was Lecturer in the Economics of the EEC. I was given the summer to prepare my teaching and so started work in July 1978. I duly turned up at 9 am on 1 July to find...no-one there. I went to the library and returned to the department every hour, and eventually went home defeated at 3 pm. I later found out. my colleagues were on holiday, or working at home, or in a library outside Edgbaston.

My first six months at Edgbaston brought me into conflict with the administrators. The department, and my mail, teaching and secretarial assistance were located on the ground in one of a pair of 'temporary' huts in the middle of the campus but I was allocated an office on the 11th floor of the University Tower. This was logistical madness but the administration refused to budge until Easter. I shared an office with my head of department on alternate days until they finally did give way. Even then, the administrators probably had the last laugh. They did allocate me an office in the huts but it had been the lost property office and had bars on the windows and a stable-type door, and it took a further six months for them to remove these and convert my office into a normal one. On the plus side, I was never lost for an umbrella or a scarf, and I was able to supplement my salary by selling walking sticks and glasses to the university health centre.

Returning to the family, Clare continues to work as a musician in Scotland in spite of her health problems and is now living in Glasgow with her boyfriend. He is a singer, currently doing a Master's in opera, who has been very supportive during her illness. I do wonder where her musical ability comes from. I can't play a musical instrument to save my life. They tried to get me to play a recorder during my first two years at secondary school but it was a lost cause from the very beginning. Anne is much the same. Nevertheless, I love Christmas music and I do not feel Christmassy until I have sung 'O Little Town of Bethlehem' at least once. I particularly like the quiet verse:

How silently, how silently,
The wondrous gift is given.
So God imparts to human hearts,
The blessings of His heaven.
No ear may hear His coming,
But in this world of sin,
Where meek souls will receive him still,
The dear Christ enters in.

Whatever happened to the meek, weren't they supposed to inherit the earth?

Merry Christmas!

Here's hoping for a better 2018!

NOVEMBER 2018

Dear

Well, Christmas approaches once again and I find myself reflecting on a year dominated by my health. It began with Christmas Day itself, a very adult affair for us with the youngest person there aged 25. This matched my mood which was one of discomfort as I was wearing a back brace and doing Hunchback of Notre Dame impersonations. First, to update you with news of my health, particularly my back problem, I did get the all clear on my back in early January 2018 and no longer had to wear a brace. I now suffer from a little back pain but it is fairly minimal. My main concerns are my walking and talking, both of which are poor. Anne is encouraging me to invest in one of those mobility scooters. I am a bit concerned as I am already a danger to vehicles and pedestrians with just a walking stick. I dread to think what sort of havoc I might create with a motorised vehicle.

In fact, I spent much of the first half of 2018 trying to reduce the chances of getting yet another disease – diabetes. They calculate a score based on various indicators:

(a score of) 40 or less: you are fine and unlikely to get diabetes;

41-47: you are "pre-diabetic" - that is, at risk and very likely to get diabetes if you don't do something about it – all the people on the course were initially within this range;

48+: you have diabetes.

The course was intensive and thorough and covered everything to do with diet and exercise. Believe me, I was worn out after the first session – a two hour lecture on fats – and had to have a huge sausage sandwich afterwards to recover. I'd no idea that fat came in so many shapes, sizes and types. It was all too much for one course participant who found a foolproof way to avoid getting diabetes when he died a few days later. It seemed a bit extreme to me. Of course, the trouble with this sort of course is that the speakers tend to be a little evangelical and assume that you will be able to spend four hours preparing breakfast and resist the temptation to eat a bacon butty and two packets of custard creams. In truth, I lacked the commitment to do the programme properly and so I approached my individual six-month review with some trepidation. But this was misplaced – in fact, I sailed through with a score of 38 – initially it was 43 - and a weight loss of just over a stone.

Still on health (sort of) – my youngest daughter, Lizzie, ran the Brighton Marathon for PD in the summer (or thereabouts). Whilst I appreciated the effort and enjoyed the day, I still tend to the view that marathon runners are a bunch of lunatics who failed to notice the discovery of the wheel and have no concept of bus timetables. In addition, Clare, my middle daughter, organised and played in a concert (for PD) along with her fiancé – yes, she is going to be married next year. It is a marriage made in musical heaven – her husband to be is an opera singer and his two siblings both musicians. That's one down and two more (daughters) to go although Angie is moving in the opposite direction, having split up with her partner.

My year with regard to my health then dropped to an all time low in the middle of the year - it has not been a good year for me. Towards the end of June pains in a longstanding hernia led to a fast ambulance ride to Worcester hospital and quick operation to sort out the problem. I found that it is absolutely terrifying to be hurtling along in an ambulance with the siren wailing and the lights flashing, clinging on for dear life every time that you turned a corner. However, I did show true British spirit when I woke up after the operation on the day of England's third World Cup match (against Belgium) and asked not about my operation but rather said: "Have England kicked off yet?" I actually came around in intensive care on a life support machine – I don't recommend it at home – and I was to lose the whole of July (and the heatwave) and was eventually to spend almost seven weeks in hospital. I also lost nearly three stones in weight and suffered from a whole range of illnesses and conditions; the weight loss was due to my stopping eating on the grounds that my food was being pureed and I refuse to eat anything that looks like a cowpat. Many of the diseases that I was afflicted by I caught in hospital. Consequently, I now have a much more negative attitude to spending time in hospital than I have expressed in earlier letters.

And the hospital had the full range of loonies and shouters - mostly people with dementia, to be politically correct. In fact, looking back, to my horror, I realise that I was one of the loonies for the first few days. But, thereafter I was definitely a spectator and listener to these poor souls although they were pretty annoying when it came to sleeping. I had the two extremes on my penultimate night – in front of me, Rambling Sid - a Manchester United fan who lived on a different planet and talked to imaginary people continuously; to my side, Mr Nasty who spent his time trying to get out of bed and (loudly) verbally-abusing the staff. This went on all night. Then there was Minnie the Screamer, the Wandering Pole and Mrs. Apparently Nice, amongst others. I don't know how the staff put up with it – but they do. Actually, I don't know how I managed to put up with it and so I'll spare you the ordeal and not talk about it anymore – although one thought does still haunt me – some of the poor devils are probably still there, talking to the walls.

That's enough misery for one letter – and now on to the real news of 2018 and the reason you are getting your Christmas card a bit early this year. After five years of reorganising and rewriting, I have finally had a collection of my letters published;

THE ALTERNATIVE CHRISTMAS LETTERS was published on 2 September (my 65th birthday).

I am not sure how much of the book you would recognise. As I've said, the original letters have been revised, edited, rearranged and extended by new material so much that you may wish to get your own copy; also you may not have been on the mailing list since the very beginning (1998).

Or you may wish to send a copy of the book to a friend or two as a Christmas present.

Or you may wish to review the book (or know someone who will) in which case could you please send the name and contact details of the reviewer and where the review will be published to me by email.

Anne was keen to celebrate my book and hospital release and so she took me to a funeral. It was that of a neighbour's mother who I'd never met at a church some miles away which we eventually found more through luck than intention. Getting into the church did not prove easy either and then just as we'd settled, I realised that I needed the toilet – desperately. In the absence of a policeman, ask a priest and so we did and I was hurriedly part-carried, part-wheelchaired and part-frog marched to a toilet behind the altar by a combination of Anne and two priests. The toilet was very small and so Anne – but not the priests – came in with me and she was suitably horrified when I pulled down my pants and produced not a number 1 but a substantial number 2. Things got even worse when I got up to leave and revealed a sign that said "Septic Tank – number 1s only and a small amount of paper. Definitely no number 2s." Anne hit the roof - or would have done, had there been room. Then we opened the door and nearly tripped over two red-faced priests, stood waiting patiently by my wheelchair, who had heard everything. We then embarked on a mad rush to get back to our seats before the coffin got to the altar. There was a real chance that we would arrive at the altar at the same time and that I, half-carried by two priests, would be mistaken for the body that had somehow got out of the coffin and was denying its death. Fortunately, we won the race and the service went well enough but my embarrassment was not yet over. You need to be reminded of two things at this point: first, there was a buffet afterwards (to which we went) and, second, I had lost three stones in weight in hospital. What you won't realise is how these apparently harmless pieces of information can combine to give surprising results. Specifically, my trousers fell down – not once but twice – and right in the middle of the main room being used for the buffet on the second occasion. By this stage, some of the other guests had begun to regard me as a kind of black/dark comedic cabaret in poor taste and so we retreated home.

Finally – well, nearly - and in a similar vein, I bring to your attention two newspaper headlines that I saw while in hospital:

- The first appeared on as a headline on p. 1 of the Worcester News and is beyond bizarre: "Give me an old ambulance …. so I can whisk my one-legged wife off to Blackpool, says Romeo OAP." It transpires that he also wants someone to donate a caravan so that he can use parts of it to convert the ambulance and that he thinks that the hospital should give him the ambulance for free as compensation for the more negative aspects of the treatment he recently received there. It seems to me that this one-legged wife is married to a one-armed bandit and they face a long lonely hop along the Golden Mile.

- I forget the precise location of the second headline but, as I recollect, it was based on an interview with Bin Laden's mother who essentially argued that her son was a good boy really who fell in with a bad crowd. The mind boggles. By the same token, was Jack the Ripper a good boy until he fell in with some bad boys who liked playing with knives!

(Definitely) finally, I ought to add one more thing about the book by reminding you that 'The Alternative Christmas Letters' like puppies and kittens, is not just for Christmas. The book is still a good read (and easy to dip in and out of) at Easter, on a beach while on holiday in the summer or on a long gloomy autumnal train journey or just in front of the fire with a steaming hot mug of drinking chocolate on a freezing winter evening. It is also not a bloody nuisance like a cat or dog which refuse to sit still on a bookshelf (unless dead or unconscious) and keep making a mess on your best carpet if you don't let them out frequently (unless dead or unconscious). So, forget that puppy or kitten and make a pet of the book. It is so much easier to look after – it doesn't need to be taken for walkies, doesn't scratch the furniture, can fend for itself when you are away and doesn't fight with other books.

On that note, I wish you a happy Christmas and a hospital-free new year!

NOVEMBER 2019

Dear

Another Christmas past and another old year nearly gone, another Christmas future and another new year will soon follow. The new millennium is now nearly 20 years old and yet it only seems like yesterday that we were worrying about what would happen to our computers at midnight on new years eve 1999 and were out strolling by the river in a sea of smiling faces at 12.15am. The sky was ablaze with fireworks and everyone was happy (presumably because their computers were still working). Of course, in those days, we actually talked to each other. Nowadays, people are glued to their smart phones watching a "live" broadcast of Big Ben chiming out midnight whilst texting "happy new year" to their nearest and dearest, stood six feet away.

We've never celebrated New Year very much in our house. When the kids were young we used to do a special meal and eat very late but can no longer be bothered. New year's resolutions are also something that I don't get involved in.

People are so unoriginal – choosing resolutions like giving up smoking or losing weight. Three questions occur to me:

1. Why are resolutions nearly always about denying yourself a pleasure - usually cigarettes, alcohol or food? Why not do the whole lot in one go and just resolve to be bloody miserable and bad tempered for the foreseeable future. Or, why not give up something that you are indifferent to (orange squash), don't/can't do anyway (juggling) or, best of all, actually dislike (carpentry, broccoli, listening to Cilla Black records or being hit with a stick).

2. Why are new year resolutions always negative – why can't they be positive? For example, why not resolve to eat at least one packet of biscuits every day or to get drunk every Friday.

3. And, crucially, why should a commitment (taken on in a drunken daze at 3am on what happens to be the first day of the year) to do something that you've already tried and failed to do be any more likely to be successful than your original attempt?

It seems to me that if my suggestions were followed then you would be much more likely to realise your resolutions and it would also free up early January for smoking, drinking and eating. This would not apply to Anne who continues to go regularly to Slimming World meetings and is likely to do so for the foreseeable future - she was recently asked to calculate her weight loss each week on average for the last eight weeks and discovered that she had lost exactly one ounce per week. At that rate it will only take another four years to lose a stone!

Just as the new year seems to bring on a desire to change something in your life so does retirement. I am actually about to enter my tenth year of retirement and have so far managed to steer clear of bungee jumping, climbing mountains, running marathons or any other stupid things that people seem to feel a need to do when they retire. Of course, retirement does leave you with little reason to get up in the morning and an incentive to vegetate. However, I think that vegetation gets an unjustifiably bad press. There is much to be said in its favour: it is relaxing and cheap, and it fills in the time nicely until the next meal or reality television show. In general, I see no reason why retired people should be more active than they were before they retired. In particular, I do not understand this obsession with gardening. What makes people think that they magically develop green fingers at the age of retirement? I hated gardening before I retired and continue to hate it since I retired. My only gardening skills are in what I call preventative gardening – that is, killing things. So, I'm good at mowing lawns and weeding, but I'm useless at everything else. In fact, to my mind, winter is the best time of the year in the garden because everything stops growing.

Turning to medical matters – yes, here comes a dull bit - I spent quite a lot of time at the local hospice this year – not practising for my demise but attending as a day patient. This was a splendid day out involving transport to and from the hospice, physiotherapy, exercise classes, a massage, reading the papers, and an excellent lunch with a choice from no less than seven sweets. I even got my hair cut and my beard trimmed one week. It was a good, busy day and also gave Anne a break (although I now regard all physiotherapists as sadists). In addition, there was a doctor and priest available. I also joined the men's group although I found the first meeting of this disconcerting - all those smiling faces jumping out from all over the place to say hello. This excessive display of cheerfulness was just too much – we were in a hospice, for goodness sake – you are supposed to be miserable, not bloody cheerful. In fact, I now know that you don't have to be miserable in a hospice and I attend Men's Space, as it is called, regularly.

Unfortunately, it was around this time that I was given a new drug which contained an ingredient which did not mix at all well with my Parkinson's drugs. The net result was that Anne came downstairs one morning to find me on the floor in the kitchen, freezing cold, unable to get up and talking nonsense. She called an ambulance and I was admitted to (Worcester) hospital. I remember nothing of this and very little of the next three days as I continued to hallucinate and inhabit my own little world. Eventually, they took me off the offending drug, and I emerged immediately from my hallucinatory world, having not slept at all for three days. It was a very strange experience – something like what taking a hallucinatory drug would be like, I imagine. At least I was only in hospital for a week. I also had an overnight stay in the QE in Birmingham to have the battery that powers my brain stimulator changed.

Moving on, the main event of the year was Clare's wedding which went very well. The wedding was about music and friends as Clare decided only to invite immediate family so that she could invite more friends. It was also quite a Scottish wedding – which was a bit strange really given that the bride and groom were from Worcester and (near)

Blackpool respectively but this didn't stop them from having plenty of guests in kilts, a piper to pipe them in and out of church and a ceilidh in the evening. They were married at Glasgow Cathedral, next to the Necropolis, the famous Glasgow graveyard. It is normally difficult to get the cathedral but Clare's fiancé has been a member of the choir for eight years and so not only did they have no trouble booking the cathedral but got the services of the choir free – most of the choir came to the wedding anyway. The best man also sang – he is an opera singer. And another professional singer whom Clare plays gigs with sang at the reception. As I've said, it was a very musical wedding.

Given that I find walking and speaking difficult, my son, James helped me out with my duties. Firstly, he walked Clare down the aisle and I took over just in front of the altar and gave her away; then at the reception, he also gave my speech (that I had written) which went very well, helped by James's performance. The groom and best man also gave excellent speeches. The two bridesmaids were Clare's two sisters and the food was very good. The day finished off with the ceilidh which allowed the men in kilts to jump about a lot – though one of them got too carried away and hurled a girl too enthusiastically across the floor and she fell and broke her elbow and ended up in A&E. Nevertheless, all-in-all, everyone had a great time. Even my 6yo grandson joined in the dancing and I was looking forward to a chance to dance the Gay Gordon or, as many of Clare's friends are gay (being mainly actors or musicians), possibly to dance with Gay Gordon. But I didn't see him and so, instead, I sat and drank whisky with two of my ex-flatmates from my undergraduate days 45 years ago who both attended Anne and I's wedding, one of them as best man.

My father-in-law also went to the wedding. He was 96 in October and is getting on very well considering he has had two strokes this year and now has heart failure. He is no longer allowed to drive (which is probably a good thing) but continues to visit us regularly on the train and gets around in Bristol on a mobility scooter. He is lucky to have very good neighbours who keep an eye on him, feed him on Sundays and look after his cat when he visits us. Turning to my unmarried children, Angie has returned to work part-time (as a care assistant); Lizzie has now got her feet on the property ladder and her partner is doing amazing things to their garden; meanwhile James also now works part-time as he has begun a part-time Master's degree at Birmingham University.

Finally, I've been following the recent floods closely. Unusually, Worcester was barely affected. On the other hand, my home town (Doncaster) certainly was. Particularly affected - in fact, completely under water- was the appropriately named village of Fishlake which is barely two miles from where I grew up. I still have a number of relatives that live in the area, including my sister, but none of them were directly affected by the floods.

So, I approach Christmas 2019 in a good frame of mind which is more than I can say for the country. Firstly, we have the floods and a general election to get through and then we still have to resolve Brexit. I think that the peace and good will associated with Christmas is sorely needed this year. And a bottle of whisky for everyone to help us cope with the floods and the election wouldn't go amiss. It won't stop us getting wet or make the choice of politician any easier but, after drinking the bottle of whisky, the floods won't seem so bad and you won't care who wins the election!

So, as is usual at this time of year, we wish you………..

A merry Christmas and a happy new year!

JULY 2020

Dear

Well what a year 2020 has been. We began with those incredible floods – almost of biblical proportions – and yet we have virtually forgotten how bad it was. The people I feel most sorry for are those who were flooded out and then had to face the coronavirus. How are you supposed to self-isolate when your home is under water? The floods just seemed to go on and on but Anne and I still managed a trip to Glasgow to see Clare. It wasn't too bad although it did involve a walk to the bridge and then a bus ride over it on the way there and a detour to and additional change of train at Stafford on the way back. However, there was some bad news for the citizens of Hereford as their swimming pool closed for two months because of flooding – no, I don't understand it either – and for cricketers and jockeys as Worcestershire's New Road ground was yet again under water, as was the racecourse; I think that I've already said before (in a previous letter), that they call it "heavy going".

Then we had the coronavirus pandemic. I've actually been

to Wuhan – I went and spoke at the first conference of the Chinese (academic) Association for EU Studies, held at Wuhan in 1993. It was a strange experience. I knew some of the delegates from a previous visit to Beijing but spent most of my time with a well-known academic (author of the leading textbook on the economics of the EU), in a grim hostel on the campus of the University. The campus was enormous but very shabby and grey. He was the only other Briton there and had recently moved from Leeds to Fukuoka in Japan. We spent most of the three days before the conference started wandering around looking for a bar and trying to get the hostel to supply us with bigger towels; we were successful in the former but not the latter.

On the first day of the conference I found myself next to a mild mannered, non-English speaking Italian who turned out to be no less than Paulo Cecchini of the Cecchini Report fame (which is the short, popular version of the European Commission's study of the gains of creating a single market in the EU). Why on earth he was there, I have no idea. Also, there was the European Commission's delegation to China, flown in from Beijing, who (wisely) opted to stay in a hotel off campus. I interviewed its (German) head for research purposes at the airport on the way home; he clearly hated being in China. We were only taken into Wuhan city centre once – to go shopping – it was as shabby and depressing as the campus. I don't blame the coronavirus for wanting to get out and see the world although the city is presumably modernised now and full of skyscrapers. (Added later: indeed it is – I've seen Wuhan recently on television.)

The whole coronavirus episode has been like a bad but - nonetheless frightening - science fiction film. We were very lucky that the beginning of the crisis coincided with the start of spring and the onset of longer, lighter evenings and actually killed relatively few people. I shudder to think what would have happened if the virus had been much more deadly and had wiped out large numbers of the population. Furthermore, what if it had started in September/October and the lights had gone out (due to the higher demand for electricity caused by people being self-isolating at home). Locking down in the cold and dark with winter on the way would not have been a lot of fun.

The lock down hasn't bothered me a great deal as I don't go out much anyway but I think that James has got a bit fed up of being at home with his parents. There is also a limit to how long you can spend sorting out your books, DVDs and clothes before boredom sets in. Anne got very bored and eventually resorted to painting the sheds and complaining incessantly about her lack of tools. I keep telling her that she ought to carry her Black and Decker around in her handbag but she won't have it.

It is truly amazing how many different groups are affected by the virus. I'd like to argue the case for bank robbers – they can't work from home and are not eligible for any furlough payments. So, they have to carry on robbing banks and this has a number of drawbacks:

1. With everyone wearing facemasks its quite difficult to differentiate between the general public and other bank robbers. This can cause practical problems if two or more gangs target the same bank.
2. If you are self-isolating your choice of accomplice

may be limited. You may have to take one of your children as a getaway driver.

3. Queuing at 2 metre intervals to go into a bank slows everything down and, with everyone wearing a mask when a robber finally reaches the counter and says "Stick'em up" he is likely not be taken seriously and may be met with a comment such as: "Congratulations you're the 100th person to crack that joke, today."

4. Your getaway is very constrained in the sense of where you can get away to. It is not always easy to hide in a park or supermarket queue wearing a black and white striped jumper and carrying a bag with 'Swag' written on it.

On the other hand, it's much easier to blend in with the crowd when everyone is wearing masks and bank robbers no longer have to fear identity parades.

Also, besides robbers, spare a thought for trapeze artistes and for those using a tandem (to avoid travelling on public transport) trying to obey the 2 metre rule. On an (even) lighter note, thank goodness for the Belarus FA. Belarus was the only country in the world to continue to play football during the crisis. The authorities denied that coronavirus had any relevance to football and, at one point, came close to denying it had any effect on Belarus at all. So the season began as usual in March and the Belarusians probably continued to insist that the earth was flat, that the Americans did not really land men on the moon in 1969, that the sun went around the earth (rather than vice versa) and that Donald Trump was a good guy who cared passionately about the future of Belarus – all of these are about as likely as the virus bypassing Belarus. I was just happy to get my fix of tv football via watching Belarus football on the internet. I soon adopted a team – FK Slutsk – who were second (after three games) in Belarus's premier league (but fell away badly afterwards).

The lack of football has been a real hardship for many men, all around the world and, starved of their football, they have taken to following Belarusian football and in particular, FK Slutsk, because of the team's amusing name. It was rumoured that the club was negotiating a sponsorship deal with a website that sold pornography. The advertising boards and players' shirts would be quite different to what we are used to.

SECTIONS ON THE AUGUST- DECEMBER PERIOD TO BE WRITTEN LATER.

I'd like to finish with an item that appeared in the Sky (online) news on 14/04/2020:

A 64-year-old man reluctantly agreed to accept a gift from colleagues of a surprise flight in a military jet, only to accidentally eject himself from the aircraft as it hurtled through the sky at 2,500ft. (Now that is really voting with your feet.) He had never expressed any desire to travel in a fighter jet, … [nor had he shown any other signs of insanity]… but he felt he had to accept the gift because his colleagues had gone to a great deal of trouble to arrange it. Nevertheless, he was said to have screamed with fear during the ordeal although he escaped injury as the ejector seat did its job efficiently. He apparently triggered the ejector catch accidentally while trying to grab something to steady himself with as the jet travelled at 320mph. The pilot went on to land the plane safely and ask if it was something he said or was the man just trying to open the window because he was too hot. (Oh, alright, I made the last bit up.)

With friends like that then who needs enemies (or, perhaps better, enemas).

Happy landings!!

Merry Christmas

POSTSCRIPT

That's all folks. You've just read a cross-section of my life over the last 20 years ago or so, a fairly ordinary life really but not without its moments of interest. The book is highly selective in its choice of moments and takes a few liberties with the truth but, on the whole it is truthful or at least, very close to being so. What is truthful history anyway? Everyone has a different interpretation of events. A potentially bigger problem is inaccurate memories. Indeed, my wife, I forget her name, insists my memory is so bad I get most things wrong. She may well be right up to a point but I don't think a few honest mistakes matter. I prefer to think of my writing as being as honest and truthful as it can reasonably be expected to be. In fact, I intend to be brutally open in my 2021 letter and include stuff that I kept out of my earlier letters – the sex, the drinking binges, the wild parties, the drugs and the bank robberies. It's a pity I won't finish it in time to include in this book. More generally, health permitting, I hope to continue to write and send my Christmas letters for a few more years yet and have added two full letters and one half-completed letter to this second edition.

It remains a source of no little surprise to me that the Christmas letter, even without the juicy bits, carries on thriving as people continue to feel the need to pass on details of the activities of their offspring, their holidays and their home improvements. We still receive some four or five of these every year and they are still quite readable. The one we get from an old friend of mine, who shall remain nameless but lives in Nottingham, is always a particularly good read. And the letter we get from Preston also deserves an honourable mention. In fact, if I have learnt anything from writing my letters, it is that Christmas letters will inevitably include material most people don't find particularly interesting. This is not a fault, it is an attribute. I succumb to this when I talk about my family and my health.

Consequently, the longevity of the Christmas letter is perhaps not that surprising, after all. So, let this book not be a complete parody and condemnation of the good old Christmas letter but be an indulgent, if critical, celebration of this particular genre of literature – an indulgent uncle rather than an angry father. In any case, I am hardly in a position to criticise other people and pass judgement on what they choose to pass on in their Christmas correspondence. I too have my failings and on a grand scale. I've never been able to decide which way the deckchair of life should face because I've never managed to put the deckchair up.

So, to bring things to an end, may all your Christmases be joyful, and may the rest of your year be pretty good as well.

Peace be with you.

Nil desperandum.

And I shall finish with the words of an excited Polish priest with limited English language skills who, overcome by the occasion at the end of one particular midnight mass on Christmas Eve, ended the service with the following words:

Happy Easter!!

ALSO BY JOHN REDMOND

The EEC and the UK Economy London: Longman: 1987

The External Relations of the European Community: The International Response to 1992 London: Macmillan: 1992

The Next Mediterranean Enlargement: Turkey, Cyprus and Malta? Aldershot: Dartmouth: 1993

Prospective Europeans London: Prentice-Hall: 1995

From Versailles to Maastricht: International Organisation in the Twentieth Century (with J. D. Armstrong and L. Lloyd) London: Macmillan: 1996

The 1995 Enlargement of the European Union London: Ashgate: 1997

Enlarging the European Union: Past, Present and Future (with

Glenda Rosenthal) Boulder, Colorado, USA: Lynne Rienner: 1998

The Enlargement of Europe (with S, Croft, W. Rees and M. Webber) Manchester: Manchester University Press: 1999

Enlarging the European Union: The Way Forward (with Jackie Gower) Aldershot: Dartmouth: 2000

International Organisation in World Politics (with J. D. Armstrong and Lorna Lloyd) London: Palgrave Macmillan: 2004

The Alternative Christmas Letters (available from Amazon): 2018

THE QUIZZES THAT NEVER WERE
(USED)

The first quiz (about Christmas) was sent as part of two letters and is therefore reproduced in the main body of the book. This section of the book is concerned with the second, third and fourth quizzes. I've been working on them on and off for a few years and they never did find their way into an actual letter, but I've finally finished them for inclusion in this book. You need a quizmaster for this one as the questions and answers, and sometimes relevant comments, are given on the same page.

QUIZ-2
WHO ARE/WERE THEY? – Q&A

Here are the real names of 25 famous people (lower case), mostly still here but some no longer with us. But what is the stage name (UPPER CASE) under which they are actually known? For example, the stage name of Harry Webb is CLIFF RICHARD.

SECTION 1 — FIVE HOLLYWOOD LEGENDS:

1. Marion Morrison - JOHN WAYNE
2. Norma Mortenson - MARILYN MONROE
3. Camille Javal - BRIGETTE BARDOT
4. Archibald Leach - CARY GRANT
5. Allen Konigsberg - WOODY ALLEN

SECTION 2 – FIVE BRITISH COMEDIANS OR ACTORS KNOWN FOR PLAYING A PARTICULAR (COMIC) TV CHARACTER.

6. John Bartholomew - ERIC MORECOMBE
7. Jim Moir - VIC REEVES
8. Michael Smith - MICHAEL CRAWFORD
9. David White - DAVID JASON
10. David Williams - DAVID WALLIAMS

SECTION 3 - TEN ESTABLISHED POP/ROCK STARS:

11. David Jones (NOT the one in the Monkees) - DAVID BOWIE
12. Gordon Sumner - STING
13. Reg Dwight - ELTON JOHN
14. William Perks – Rolling Stones bass player - BILL WYMAN
15 Richard Starkey - RINGO STARR
16. Vincent Furnier - ALICE COOPER

17. Paul Hewson - BONO
18. Priscilla White - CILLA BLACK
19. Robert Zimmerman - BOB DYLAN
20. David Cook - DAVID ESSEX

SECTION 4 - POT POURRI

FIVE questions of which the first three are a model, an iconic retired footballer and a doctor (not necessarily in that order);

And the last two are pen names of famous authors used for all his books in one case and for just a few books in the other after she had already become famous as a writer under her own name.

21. David McDonald - DAVID TENNANT
22. Lesley Hornby - TWIGGY
23. Edson Arantes do Nascimento - PELE
24. Eric Blair - GEORGE ORWELL
25. Robert Galbraith - J. K. ROWLING

QUIZ-3
HISTORY OF FOOTBALL - Q&A
(DIFFICULT)

FOOTBALL QUIZ FOR MEN WHO CAN REMEMBER WHEN THERE WAS NO PREMIER LEAGUE AND KEVIN KEEGAN HADN'T HAD A PERM

-A- FOOTBALL PLAYERS (5 points)

-1- Who is generally regarded as the country's first £100,000 player? (1)

JIMMY GREAVES (From AC Milan to Tottenham Hotspur in 1961).

-2- Which Northern comic (from Barnsley) played 171 times for Doncaster Rovers in the early 1950s? (1)

CHARLIE WILLIAMS

-3- Bobby Moore lifted a trophy each year at Wembley in 1964-65-66. Name all three trophies and indicate in which year each of them were won. (1)

1964 (FA CUP), 1965 (EUROPEAN CUP WINNERS CUP) AND 1966 (WORLD CUP)

-4- Two of the 1966 England World Cup squad played for Blackpool but only one of them actually played in the final. Can you name either of them? (1)

ALAN BALL played in the final, JIMMY ARMFIELD didn't

-5- Which 1960s striker was nicknamed the "King" by the fans of his club? (1)

DENIS LAW

-B- FOOTBALL CLUBS (MULTIPLE ANSWERS) (15 points)

-6/7- As well as Celtic and Rangers, there are two other teams based in Glasgow. Name them. (a point for each) (2)

PARTICK THISTLE AND QUEEN'S PARK

-8/9- Two of the early (but not founder) members of the Football League were Small Heath and Newton Heath. Both these clubs changed their name. What have they become? (a point for each) (2)

SMALL HEATH BECAME BIRMINGHAM CITY.
NEWTON HEATH BECAME MANCHESTER UNITED.

-10/11/12- The football league kicked off on 8 September 1888 with just 12 clubs. Can you name 3 of them? (a point for each) (3)

ANY THREE OF:

ACCRINGTON

ASTON VILLA

BLACKBURN ROVERS

BOLTON WANDERERS

BURNLEY

DERBY COUNTY

EVERTON

NOTTS COUNTY

PRESTON NORTH END

STOKE (CITY FROM 1926)

WEST BROMWICH ALBION

WOLVERHAMPTON WANDERERS

-13/14/15- Which 3 English clubs did Gary Lineker play for? (a point for each) (3)

LEICESTER CITY, TOTTENHAM HOTSPURS AND EVERTON.

-16/17/18/19/20- Here are 5 clubs with their present grounds Where did they play previously? (a point for each answer) (5)

Arsenal: (Emirates Stadium) - HIGHBURY

Manchester City: (City of Manchester Stadium) – MAINE ROAD

Leicester City: (King Power Stadium) – FILBERT STREET

Sunderland: (Stadium of Light) – ROKER PARK

Middlesbrough: (Riverside Stadium) – AYRESOME PARK

-C- FOOTBALL CUPS AND TROPHIES (5 points)

-21- Name the first British club to win the European Cup? (1)

CELTIC BEAT INTER MILAN 2-1 IN LISBON IN 1967.

-22- In what decade was the first ever World Cup held? (1)

THE 1930s. (1930 IN URUGUAY, 1934 IN ITALY, 1938 IN FRANCE AND THEN NOT UNTIL 1950 IN BRAZIL)

-23- The 1966 World Cup was held in England but where were the World Cups immediately before (1962) and after (1970) held? (a point for either answer) (1)

1962 – CHILE

1970 – MEXICO

-24 - The FA Cup has only been won by a non-English team once. Who was it and in what decade did it happen? (a point for either answer) (1)

THE 1920S AND CARDIFF CITY.

(IN 1927, TWO YEARS AFTER THEY HAD BEEN BEATEN FINALISTS, CARDIFF CITY DEFEATED THE MUCH FANCIED ARSENAL 1-0. THE MATCH WAS DECIDED BY A BIZARRE OWN GOAL SCORED BY THE ARSENAL GOALKEEPER, DAN LEWIS, WHO COINCIDENTALLY WAS A WELSH INTERNATIONAL, HAVING MADE HIS DEBUT FOR WALES IN FEBRUARY 1927.

-25- What was so special about the 1953 Cup Final? (1)

IT WAS KNOWN AS 'THE STANLEY MATTHEWS FINAL' WHEN MATTHEWS, THEN AGED 38, FINALLY GOT HIS FA CUP WINNER'S MEDAL AS BLACKPOOL BEAT BOLTON 4-3.

QUIZ – 4
EUROPE – Q&A

SECTION 1 - TWENTIETH CENTURY HISTORY

-1- In which European country was there a civil war in the second half of the 1930s?

SPAIN (THE SPANISH CIVIL WAR RAN FROM 1936 TO 1939.)

-2- WWII was prompted by the German invasion of Poland but Italy invaded another country even earlier (in 1935). Name the country.

ABYSSINIA (ETHIOPIA)

-3- Coventry was badly bombed in WW2. What is generally regarded as the equivalent city in Germany which suffered a similar fate?

DRESDEN

-4- The Russians sent tanks into Czechoslovakia in 1968 to maintain Soviet domination. To what country did they do more or less the same in 1956?

HUNGARY

-5- What year did the Berlin wall come down?

1989

SECTION 2 – PLACES AND PEOPLE

-6- Why was Notre Dame Cathedral in Paris in the news in 2019?

IT WAS BADLY DAMAGED BY A FIRE

-7- In what country is Valetta?.

VALETTA IS THE CAPITAL OF MALTA

-8- Who famously vetoed Britain's two applications to join the EU in the 1960s?

PRESIDENT OF FRANCE, GENERAL CHARLES DE GAULLE

-9- Andorra is the sixth smallest nation in Europe – but where is it? Name both the countries with which it has a border.

FRANCE AND SPAIN. (IT IS IN THE EASTERN PYRENEES).

-10- Which British politician is the only Briton to have been the president of the European Commission (1977-81)?

ROY JENKINS

SECTION 3 - SPORT

-11- Which football club has been the champions of Europe (by winning the Champions League or its predecessor, the European Cup) on the most occasions.

REAL MADRID

-12- England, Wales, Scotland, Ireland, France and Italy all qualified for the final stages of the 2019 rugby union world cup held in Japan. So did two other European countries. For one point name one of them.

RUSSIA OR GEORGIA.

-13- Since the Ryder Cup became a contest between the USA and Europe in 1979 which team has won the most times – the USA or Europe?

EUROPE (PRIOR TO THE 2020 CONTEST, THE STANDINGS WERE EUROPE 11, USA 8, WITH 1 TIED.)

-14- Which female, European tennis player has won more Wimbledon ladies single titles than any other European since the open era began in 1967? (Martina Navratilova counts as an American)

STEFFI GRAF (7 TITLES)

-15- Catalan Dragons play in the English Rugby League Super League but what country are they based in?

FRANCE (PERPIGNAN)

SECTION 4 - THE EUROPEAN UNION

-16- Name three of the six founding members of the EU. (one point for all 3, no points for 2 or 1.

WEST GERMANY (GERMANY IS ACCEPTABLE THOUGH TECHNICALLY WRONG – EAST GERMANY WAS A SEPARATE COUNTRY AND DID NOT BECOME PART OF THE EU UNTIL THE BERLIN WALL CAME DOWN AND GERMANY WAS UNIFIED), FRANCE, ITALY AND THE THREE BENELUX COUNTRIES (BELGIUM, THE NETHERLANDS AND LUXEMBOURG)

-17- What is the name of the currency used by most of the members of the EU?

THE EURO

-18- Which of the following countries has NOT formally applied to join the EU at some time or other?

Morocco, Switzerland, Turkey, Iceland, Israel.

THE ANSWER IS ISRAEL. (THE OTHERS HAVE ALL APPLIED IN THE YEAR INDICATED: MOROCCO, 1987; SWITZERLAND, 1992; TURKEY, 1987; ICELAND, 2009).

-19- The European Parliament operates on three sites – in Brussels, Strasbourg and …where?

LUXEMBOURG

-20- After the UK left the EU in 2020, the EU was left with how many member states? (I'll accept answers up to three less or more.)

27 (24, 25, 26, 28, 29 or 30 is acceptable.)

SECTION 5 – POT LUCK

-21- What is Eurostar's last stop (going from the UK to France) before it enters the Channel Tunnel?

ASHFORD INTERNATIONAL (ASHFORD WILL DO)

-22- What is the longest river in Europe?

THE VOLGA - IT RUNS THROUGH CENTRAL RUSSIA INTO THE CASPIAN SEA. (THE DANUBE IS THE SECOND LONGEST.)

-23- The Baltic countries are a grouping of three small countries on the eastern coast of the Baltic Sea in Northern Europe. For one point can you name all three?

LATVIA, LITHUANIA AND ESTONIA

-24- There are four main islands in the Balearic group, all of them popular tourist destinations. For one point, name two of them.

ANY TWO OF: MAJORCA, MENORCA, IBIZA AND FORMENTERA.

-25- In 1969 the Eurovision Song Contest finished in a four-way tie. One of the joint winners was the UK. Who sang for Britain?

LULU (BOOM BANG-A-BANG)

WORK IN PROGRESS

I did not write a sequel (*Letters from a Mexican*) to the first edition of this book despite expressing an intention to do that and, indeed, quickly abandoned trying to do so. Writing in 1-2 years a second volume of a book that had evolved over 20 years proved impossible. And, as I admitted in the first edition, I know nothing about Mexico and have avoided South America in general on the grounds that I don't like the weather there, the Amazon is full of anacondas and Bear Grylls and his mates making documentaries, and all the really good Brazilian footballers are playing in the English Premier League anyway.

In fact, I wrote a comic novel instead. But I did not give up the idea of writing a sequel (see below). I cannot promise that I will deliver all the following but at the time of writing (July 2020), it is my intention to do so. You can see if I did by looking at my author's page on Amazon. I currently have four active projects at various stages:

ONE The 3-in-1 Solution

This just needs a final proofread and then it is ready to go to Amazon. It is a novel and is very different to this book – still humorous (hopefully) but with a very dark side. It is based in a university and written in my usual quirky style. It introduces Inspector Sweeper of the yard. It should be available shortly after this book appears.

TWO Sweeper Digs Deep

This is the second book in the Sweeper series and sees Sweeper investigating several bizarre deaths in a mining community. I have written the first 3,000 words.

THREE A Glitch in Time Solves Crime

This is little more than a brief plot idea which will have Sweeper investigate a murder which seems to be a copycat murder of an unsolved case in the past. It is set in the sporting world – the original crime in the world of football in the 1960s/1970s, the copycat in the world of rugby in the current period (2001-2020).

FOUR A Normal Life

This is a very straight, dull and boring autobiography which is being written for my children and is highly unlikely ever to be offered for publication. It will probably be of little interest to anyone except my close relatives anyway. I currently have about half of it lying around.

.   .   .

I have a number of other ideas for books which are little more than ideas at the moment. These include an introduction to personal finances for teenagers, a coffee table book about dead rock stars and a travel book (comparing trips to the superpowers in the late 1980s and early 1990s when I visited Beijing, Brussels, Moscow and Washington). Whether these books are displaced by new projects and/or I live long enough to write them remains to be seen.

ACKNOWLEDGMENTS

First and foremost, I would like to thank all the friends and relatives who have read and encouraged me to write my letters over the years, and I thank those of you who have retaliated in kind by sending letters to me. There are 25-30 of you out there and the feedback I have received has always been positive, which of course is not to say there isn't a silent majority who hate my letters but are too polite to say so. If this is the case, I thank you for keeping quiet. Second, I would like to thank Joe Czternastek who I have known for 45 years, probably owe money to, and who read and commented on part of the book. He also did some of the research I failed to do and corrected some of my errors.

In addition, I wish to thank my old university pal, Frank Kusy (whom I found on Amazon and re-established contact with after a gap of nearly 40 years) for his advice, encouragement and gentle introduction to the mysteries of non-academic publishing. I would also like to thank Victoria Twead of Ant Press, who completed my publishing education and saved me from the technical horrors of transforming my manuscript into an Amazon paperback, a Kindle book, and something that can be bought and read on various other platforms. Furthermore, I wish to give thanks to Liz Ellis, formerly my fellow (and now ex-) Worcester Warriors fan, who has helped me in various ways, notably by switching her allegiance to Leicester, who immediately started to lose regularly to Worcester.

Last, and most of all, my thanks go to my wife and children, to whom this book is dedicated, who have had to suffer many of the consequences of my having Parkinson's Disease, and will now have to suffer the consequences of having a husband/father who writes strange books. Moreover, they have unwittingly provided material for the book and also had, and have, to live in the situation comedy that I sometimes feel that my life has become.

ABOUT THE AUTHOR

John Redmond was born in 1953, the son, grandson and great-grandson of miners, and grew up in a South Yorkshire mining village in the 1950s and 1960s. He has lived in Worcester for the last 30 years. He graduated from the Universities of Cardiff and Warwick and lectured at the University of Birmingham for 30 years, the last thirteen of which as Professor of European Studies. He was diagnosed with Parkinson's Disease at the age of 42 in 1995 and took early retirement on ill health grounds at the age of 57 in 2010. While his career has been based on the traditional three Rs: reading, (w)riting and (a)rithmetic, his leisure has been concerned with three Rs of his own: rock music, real ale and rugby union. Inevitably, all of these interests feature to some extent in this book. He has published numerous academic books but 'The Alternative Christmas Letters' is his first foray into non-academic territory. He celebrated his 40th wedding anniversary in 2018, with the same wife he had at the beginning, and they have four children and four grandchildren.

The author's contact details can be found on the author's Author Page on Amazon.

Printed in Great Britain
by Amazon

11590140R00142